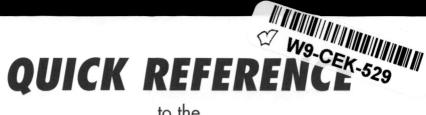

QUICK REFERENCE

to the

American Psychiatric Association

Practice Guidelines for the Treatment of Psychiatric Disorders

COMPENDIUM 2004

QUICK REFERENCE

to the

American Psychiatric Association

Practice Guidelines for the Treatment of Psychiatric Disorders

COMPENDIUM 2004

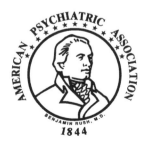

Published by the
American Psychiatric Association
Arlington, Virginia

Note: The authors have worked to ensure that all information in this book concerning drug dosages, schedules, and routes of administration is accurate as of the time of publication and consistent with standards set by the U.S. Food and Drug Administration and the general medical community. As medical research and practice advance, however, therapeutic standards may change. Moreover, specific situations may require a specific therapeutic response not included in this book. For these reasons and because human and mechanical errors sometimes occur, we recommend that readers follow the advice of a physician who is directly involved in their care or the care of a member of their family.

Copyright © 2004 American Psychiatric Association
ALL RIGHTS RESERVED
Manufactured in the United States of America on acid-free paper
07 06 05 04   4 3 2 1

American Psychiatric Association
1000 Wilson Boulevard
Arlington, VA 22209-3901
www.psych.org

Library of Congress Cataloging-in-Publication Data
American Psychiatric Association
    Quick reference to the American Psychiatric Association practice guidelines for the
treatment of psychiatric disorders, Compendium 2004.
        p. ; cm.
    Includes bibliographical references.
    ISBN 0-89042-377-6 (pbk. : alk. paper)
        I. Title: Practice guidelines for the treatment of psychiatric disorders. II. American
    Psychiatric Association. American Psychiatric Association practice guidelines for the
    treatment of psychiatric disorders, Compendium 2004. III. Title.
        [DNLM: 1. Mental Disorders—therapy—Handbooks. 2. Mental
    Disorders—diagnosis—Handbooks. WM 400 A5131a 2004 Suppl.]
    RC480.A527 2004
    616.89′1—dc22
                                                                        2003062795
British Library Cataloguing in Publication Data
A CIP record is available from the British Library.

For Continuing Medical Education credit
for APA Practice Guidelines,
visit **www.psych.org/cme.**

To order individual Practice Guidelines or the
2004 Compendium of APA Practice Guidelines,
visit **www.appi.org** or call **800-368-5777.**

The American Board of Psychiatry and Neurology (ABPN) has reviewed
the APA Practice Guidelines CME Program and has approved
this product as part of a comprehensive lifelong learning program,
which is mandated by the American Board of Medical Specialties
as a necessary component of maintenance of certification.

ABPN approval is time limited to 3 years for each individual Practice Guideline CME course.
Refer to APA's CME web site for ABPN approval status of each course.

Contents

Statement of Intent

The Practice Guidelines and the Quick Reference Guides are not intended to be construed or to serve as a standard of medical care. Standards of medical care are determined on the basis of all clinical data available for an individual case and are subject to change as scientific knowledge and technology advance and practice patterns evolve. These parameters of practice should be considered guidelines only. Adherence to them will not ensure a successful outcome in every case, nor should they be construed as including all proper methods of care or excluding other acceptable methods of care aimed at the same results. The ultimate judgment regarding a particular clinical procedure or treatment plan must be made by the psychiatrist in light of the clinical data presented by the patient and the diagnostic and treatment options available.

The development of the APA Practice Guidelines and Quick Reference Guides has not been financially supported by any commercial organization.

Introduction

This compendium contains 10 quick reference guides (QRGs), each derived from the full text of a practice guideline developed by the American Psychiatric Association (APA) and published originally in *The American Journal of Psychiatry*. One of the QRGs included (for suicidal behaviors) is new since the publication of the previous compendium, and one (for schizophrenia) has been extensively revised. A previously published QRG on substance use disorders was excluded from this compendium because the practice guideline from which it is derived was determined to be out of date; a revision is in progress. The purpose of these QRGs is to facilitate clinical use of APA's practice guidelines by physicians.

The term *practice guideline* refers to a set of patient care strategies developed to assist physicians in clinical decision making. Launched in 1989, APA's evidence-based practice guidelines project has published 13 guidelines since 1993. The project's development process has been heavily influenced by a 1990 Institute of Medicine guideline report and by the criteria for guidelines promulgated by the American Medical Association Practice Parameters Partnership. APA's guidelines have been widely acclaimed as comprehensive and scholarly documents and are increasingly being used in residency education, certification examinations, utilization review, and, most important, clinical decision making by psychiatrists.

The idea to develop QRGs for APA's practice guidelines resulted from frequent comments by psychiatrists that although the practice guidelines provide detailed recommendations for treatment and comprehensively describe the evidence to support those recommendations, their length and text format do not allow for easy use in the psychiatrist's day-to-day work with patients. Feedback of this type is not unique to the APA effort. Despite publication of a large number of well-researched and thoughtfully developed guidelines in many fields of medicine, as well as strong encouragement of medical associations and academic and opinion leaders to use guidelines, actual rates of use by clinicians have been disappointingly low. Therefore, dissemination and implementation strategies have become the major foci of guideline projects, including APA's.

The first APA QRG (on major depressive disorder) was developed in 1997 as part of a study in conjunction with RAND Corporation and the New York State Psychiatric Association, with grant support from the New York State Department of Health. The response of psychiatrists using the QRG made clear that it was indeed a helpful tool; thereafter, development of a QRG for each practice guideline became an important component of the APA practice guidelines project.

The process of constructing a QRG is as follows: Dr. Michael B. First, who became Medical Editor for the QRGs in 2000, begins by abstracting crucial information from the full guideline, which ensures that the QRG closely follows the wording of the parent guideline. The abstracted text is then shortened further, with greatest emphasis placed on material most directly relevant to treatment decision making. Thus, material about diagnosis, epidemiology, and other background information is not included. Similarly, because of constraints on length, most of the information regarding treatment for special populations is excluded. The resulting draft is reviewed by APA staff working with the practice guidelines project, including Robert Kunkle, Claudia Hart, and Dr. Laura J. Fochtmann, who provide detailed comments and edits. A second draft that incorporates these comments is reviewed for accuracy by the work group that developed the original practice guideline. Finally, the QRG is reviewed, edited, and approved by the Executive Committee for Practice Guidelines, who are Drs. John S. McIntyre, Sara C. Charles, Kenneth Altshuler, Ian Cook, Sherwyn Woods, and Joel Yager.

The main challenge in developing a QRG is to present the major recommendations and their sequencing in enough detail to be clinically helpful and at the same time to limit the document to a usable length. The initial aim was to make the QRGs shorter than they are, but the more important goal of clearly identifying key issues and recommendations necessitated a longer length. The result, we think, is comprehensive and practical.

Central to proper use of these QRGs is recognition that they do not stand alone. The psychiatrist using this QRG will find it helpful to return to the full-text practice guideline for clarification of a recommendation or for a review of the evidence supporting a particular strategy. The QRG faithfully reflects the content of the guideline, with rare exception. In the interval between development of the original practice guidelines and development of this QRG compendium, new medications became approved for use in the United States and one medication mentioned in a practice guideline as anticipating FDA approval was withdrawn. To reflect these changes, recommendations regarding medications in the QRGs for major depressive disorder and HIV/AIDS have been revised.

An essential feature of good guidelines is that they are revised at regular intervals based on advances in the knowledge base and on input from guideline users.

To date, four APA practice guidelines, on major depressive disorder, eating disorders, bipolar disorder, and schizophrenia, have been revised. As more APA practice guidelines are revised, so will be their corresponding QRGs. In addition, the Steering Committee on Practice Guidelines has begun to publish "guideline watches," brief articles that highlight new and significant scientific developments relevant to specific guidelines. At the time of publication of this compendium, watches were in development for the practice guidelines on psychiatric evaluation of adults, delirium, Alzheimer's disease and other dementias of late life, and panic disorder. As they are completed, these and other watches will be made available online on the Practice Guidelines page in the Psychiatric Practice section of the APA web site at www.psych.org. Psychiatrists who use the QRGs in this compendium are advised to check the web site periodically to stay informed about important scientific developments that may affect how they decide to implement guideline recommendations in their clinical practice.

Psychiatrists using the QRGs are encouraged to submit suggestions for improvement of these tools.

John S. McIntyre, M.D.
Chair, APA Steering Committee on Practice Guidelines

Sara C. Charles, M.D.
Vice-Chair, APA Steering Committee on Practice Guidelines

Michael B. First, M.D.
Medical Editor, Quick Reference Guides

TREATING DELIRIUM
A Quick Reference Guide

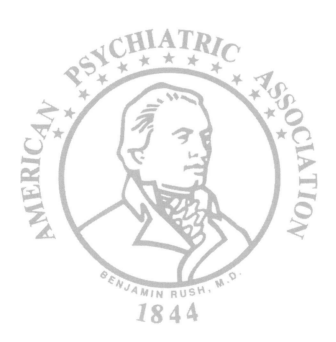

Based on *Practice Guideline for the Treatment of Patients With Delirium,*
originally published in May 1999. A guideline watch, summarizing significant developments
in the scientific literature since publication of this guideline, may be available in the
Psychiatric Practice section of the APA web site at www.psych.org.

OUTLINE

A. Diagnosis and Assessment

1. Diagnosis of Delirium

- Conduct a thorough assessment of the patient's symptoms, including all DSM-IV criteria for delirium as well as associated features of delirium (e.g., disturbances in sleep, psychomotor activity, and emotions).
- Distinguish among differential diagnostic possibilities; for patients with features of delirium, the most common issue is determining whether the patient has dementia, delirium, or both.
- Obtain information from medical records, psychiatric records, medical staff, family, and other sources.

2. Assessment of Clinical Status

Conduct a thorough assessment of the patient's clinical status, including
- the patient's potential for harm to self or others,
- the availability of means for harm to self or others and the lethality of those means, and
- the presence of hallucinations and delusions.

Evaluate comorbid general medical conditions and past medical history.
- Patients with delirium require a comprehensive evaluation of their current and past medical conditions and treatments, including medications, with special attention paid to those conditions or treatments that might be contributing to the delirium.
- Evaluation by the psychiatrist is frequently coordinated and conducted jointly with the patient's internist, neurologist, and other primary care and specialty physicians.

2. Assessment of Clinical Status (continued)

Conduct a thorough history of current patterns of alcohol and other substance use.

Conduct a thorough assessment of other current psychiatric disorders or symptoms.

Conduct a thorough assessment of the patient's past psychiatric history, including
- previous episodes of delirium,
- dangerousness to self or others,
- previous treatment responses, and
- prior alcohol and other substance use.

Conduct a thorough assessment of the patient's psychosocial history, including
- family and interpersonal relationships;
- premorbid psychosocial, work, living, and cultural environment; and
- availability of family members or other surrogates capable of helping with decision making for patients who lack decisional capacity.

Knowledge of the patient's and family's psychological and social characteristics may be helpful in dealing with the anxieties and reactions of patients and families.

B. Psychiatric Management

Throughout the formulation of a treatment plan and the subsequent course of treatment, the following principles of psychiatric management should be kept in mind:

1. Coordinate with other physicians.

Treatment of patients with delirium frequently requires joint and coordinated management among psychiatrists and other general medical and specialty physicians.

2. Identify etiological factors and correct them.

Review information from the patient's medical and psychiatric history, family members, and other individuals close to the patient.

Conduct indicated laboratory and radiological investigations to determine the underlying cause or causes of the patient's delirium. The choice of specific tests will be guided by the results of clinical evaluations and may include those outlined in Table 1 (p. 6).

3. Initiate acute interventions.

- Patients with delirium may have general medical conditions that require urgent therapeutic intervention, even before an etiology for the delirium is identified.
- Increased observation and monitoring of the patient's general medical condition are often necessary, including frequent monitoring of vital signs, fluid intake and output, and oxygenation level.

TABLE 1. Assessment of Patients With Delirium

Physical status
- History
- General physical and neurological examinations
- Review of vital signs and anesthesia record if postoperative
- Review of general medical and psychiatric records
- Careful review of medications and correlation with behavioral changes

Mental status
- Interview
- Cognitive tests (e.g., clock face, digit span, Trail Making tests)

Basic laboratory tests (consider for all patients with delirium)
- Blood chemistries: electrolytes, glucose, calcium, albumin, blood urea nitrogen (BUN), creatinine, SGOT, SGPT, bilirubin, alkaline phosphatase, magnesium, phosphorus
- Complete blood count (CBC)
- Electrocardiogram (ECG)
- Chest X-ray
- Arterial blood gases or oxygen saturation
- Urinalysis

Additional laboratory tests (order as indicated by clinical condition)
- Urine culture and sensitivity (C&S)
- Urine drug screen
- Blood tests (e.g., VDRL, heavy metal screen, B_{12} and folate levels, antinuclear antibody [ANA], urinary porphyrins, ammonia level, human immunodeficiency virus [HIV], erythrocyte sedimentation rate [ESR])
- Blood cultures
- Serum levels of medications (e.g., digoxin, theophylline, phenobarbital, cyclosporine)
- Lumbar puncture
- Brain computerized tomography (CT) or magnetic resonance imaging (MRI)
- Electroencephalogram (EEG)

Source. Adapted from Trzepacz PT, Wise MG: "Neuropsychiatric Aspects of Delirium," in *The American Psychiatric Press Textbook of Neuropsychiatry,* Third Edition. Edited by Yudofsky SC, Hales RE. Washington, DC, American Psychiatric Press, 1997, pp. 447–470.

4. Provide other disorder-specific treatments.

Reversible causes of delirium that are identified should be promptly treated as noted in Table 2 (p. 8).

5. Monitor and ensure safety.

- Monitor patients with delirium for their potential to harm themselves or others. Harmful behaviors are often inadvertent or are responses to hallucinations or delusions.
- Take appropriate measures to prevent harm to self or others. Whenever possible, the least restrictive but effective measures should be employed.

6. Assess and monitor psychiatric status.

- Regularly monitor symptoms and behaviors, as they can fluctuate rapidly.
- Adjust treatment strategies accordingly.

7. Establish and maintain alliances with patient and family.

- Establish a supportive therapeutic stance with patients.
- Establish strong alliances with the patient's family members, multiple clinicians, and caregivers.

8. Educate regarding the illness.

- Education regarding the current delirium, its etiology, and its course should be provided to patients and tailored to their ability to understand their condition.
- Education regarding delirium may also be extremely beneficial to patients' families, nursing staff, and other medical clinicians.

TABLE 2.   Examples of Reversible Causes of Delirium and
            Their Treatments

Condition	Treatment
Hypoglycemia or delirium of unknown etiology in which hypoglycemia is suspected	• Tests of blood (usually finger stick) to establish diagnosis • Thiamine hydrochloride, 100 mg i.v. (before glucose) • 50% glucose solution, 50 mL i.v.
Hypoxia or anoxia (e.g., due to pneumonia, obstructive or restrictive pulmonary disease, cardiac disease, hypotension, severe anemia, or carbon monoxide poisoning)	• Immediate oxygen
Hyperthermia (e.g., temperature above 40.5°C or 105°F)	• Rapid cooling
Severe hypertension (e.g., blood pressure of 260/150 mm Hg, with papilledema)	• Prompt antihypertensive treatment
Alcohol or sedative withdrawal	• Appropriate pharmacological intervention • Thiamine, intravenous glucose, magnesium, phosphate, and other B vitamins, including folate
Wernicke's encephalopathy	• Thiamine hydrochloride, 100 mg i.v., followed by thiamine daily, either intravenously or orally
Anticholinergic delirium	• Withdrawal of offending agent • In severe cases, physostigmine should be considered unless contraindicated

9. Provide postdelirium management.

- Following recovery, reiterate explanations to patient and family about delirium, its etiology, and its course in order to prevent recurrences.
- Provide education regarding the apparent cause or causes of and risk factors for delirium.
- Employ supportive interventions for patients experiencing distressing postdelirium symptoms.

C. Environmental and Supportive Interventions

1. Environmental Interventions

Employ environmental interventions to reduce factors that may exacerbate delirium.
These interventions include
- changing the lighting to cue day and night,
- reducing monotony and overstimulation and understimulation,
- correcting visual and auditory impairments (e.g., retrieve glasses, hearing aids), and
- rendering the patient's environment less alien by having familiar people and objects present (e.g., family photographs).

2. Structure and Support for Patients

Reorient the patient to person, place, time, and circumstances.
Reorientation should be provided by all who come into contact with the patient.

Provide reassurance to patients that the deficits they are experiencing are common but usually temporary and reversible.

3. Support and Education for Families

➤ Educate the patient's family and friends about delirium and reassure them that the patient's deficits are usually temporary and reversible.

➤ Encourage the patient's family and friends to reassure and reorient the patient and increase the familiarity of the patient's environment by increasing staff time with the patient and by bringing in familiar objects to show the patient.

D. Specific Somatic Interventions

1. Antipsychotic Medications

➤ **Haloperidol**
High-potency antipsychotic medications, such as haloperidol, are the pharmacological treatment of choice for delirium.
- Haloperidol may be administered orally, intramuscularly, or intravenously.
- Initial dosages of haloperidol are in the range of 1 to 2 mg every 2 to 4 hours, with lower starting dosages for elderly patients (e.g., 0.25 to 0.50 mg every 4 hours).
- Continuous intravenous infusion of haloperidol may be considered for severely ill patients with refractory symptoms requiring multiple bolus doses. With ECG monitoring, intravenous haloperidol can be initiated with a bolus dose of up to 10 mg followed by infusion of up to 5 to 10 mg/hour.
- When using haloperidol to treat delirium, monitor ECG. For QTc intervals greater than 450 msec or greater than 25% over baseline, consider cardiology consultation and antipsychotic medication discontinuation.

Droperidol
- Droperidol may be considered for acute agitation because of its more rapid onset of action, greater sedative properties, and shorter half-life.
- Droperidol may be administered either alone or followed by haloperidol.
- As with haloperidol, monitor ECG. Droperidol use has been associated with QTc prolongation, torsades de pointes, and sudden death.

Newer antipsychotic medications
- Risperidone, olanzapine, and quetiapine have been increasingly used to treat delirium, in part because of their more tolerable side effect profile.
- Randomized, double-blind, placebo-controlled trials of these medications in patients with delirium are not yet available.

2. Other Interventions for Delirium Caused by Specific Etiologies

Benzodiazepines
- Benzodiazepines as monotherapy are generally reserved for patients with delirium caused by seizures or withdrawal from alcohol/sedative-hypnotics.
- Benzodiazepines such as lorazepam that are relatively short acting and have no active metabolites may be preferable.
- The combination of a benzodiazepine with an antipsychotic may be a consideration for patients who can tolerate only lower doses of antipsychotic medications or who have prominent anxiety or agitation.
- Combined treatment can be initiated with 3 mg i.v. of haloperidol followed immediately by 0.5 to 1.0 mg i.v. of lorazepam.

2. Other Interventions for Delirium Caused by Specific Etiologies *(continued)*

Cholinergics
Cholinergic medications, such as physostigmine and tacrine, may be useful in delirium caused by anticholinergic agents.

Paralysis and ventilation
Agitated patients whose delirium is caused by severe hypercatabolic conditions such as hyperdynamic heart failure, adult respiratory distress syndrome, or hyperthyroid storm may require paralysis and mechanical ventilation.

Opioids
For patients with delirium in whom pain is an aggravating factor, palliative treatment with an opiate should be considered.

Vitamins
Patients with delirium at risk for B vitamin deficiency, such as alcoholic or malnourished patients, should be given multivitamin replacement.

Electroconvulsive therapy (ECT)
ECT may be a consideration in some cases of delirium caused by neuroleptic malignant syndrome. The potential benefit of ECT should be weighed against the risks of such a procedure in patients who are often medically unstable.

TREATING
ALZHEIMER'S DISEASE AND OTHER DEMENTIAS OF LATE LIFE
A Quick Reference Guide

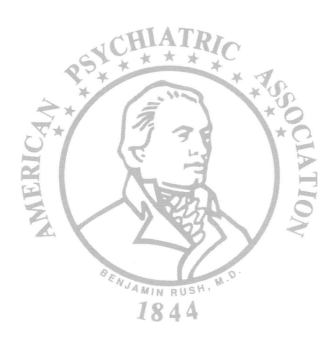

Based on *Practice Guideline for the Treatment of Patients With Alzheimer's Disease and Other Dementias of Late Life*, originally published in May 1997. A guideline watch, summarizing significant developments in the scientific literature since publication of this guideline, may be available in the Psychiatric Practice section of the APA web site at www.psych.org.

13

OUTLINE

A. Evaluation, Assessment, and Monitoring

1. Diagnostic Evaluation

Perform psychiatric, neurological, and general medical evaluations.
- Determine the nature and cause of cognitive and noncognitive symptoms.
- Identify treatable general medical conditions that may cause or exacerbate dementia.
- Provide or refer for needed medical care.

2. Assessment and Monitoring of Symptoms

Identify presence, range, and severity of symptoms.

Monitor the patient.
- Monitor cognitive and noncognitive psychiatric symptoms over the course of the illness and in response to interventions.
- Assess patients with dementia at least two to three times per year. Those who have certain symptoms (e.g., aggressive behavior) or who are undergoing specific treatments may require more frequent monitoring.

3. Safety Considerations

Assess the patient's potential for violence and suicide.

Assess adequacy of supervision.

3. Safety Considerations (continued)

Make every effort to limit the risk of falls.
- Minimize orthostatic hypotension.
- Keep medications that have CNS effects to a minimum.
- Alter environment (e.g., remove loose rugs).
- Ensure appropriate supervision while walking, toileting, etc.

Intervene to decrease the hazards of wandering.
- Advise the patient's family of danger.
- Ensure adequate supervision to prevent wandering into risky situations.
- Structure the environment to prevent unsupervised departures.
- Provide secure door locks and other methods to hinder easy exits.

Address any signs of neglect or abuse.

4. Assessment of Whether Driving Is Appropriate

Review risks of driving with the patient and his or her family.
All patients and their families should be informed that even mild dementia increases the risk of having an accident when driving or operating dangerous equipment.

Assess mildly impaired patients for a need to stop or limit driving.
See section C.1, p. 20, for a description of mild impairment.

Moderately and severely impaired patients should not drive.
- See section C.1, p. 20, for descriptions of moderate and severe impairments.
- Legal requirements for reporting impairment vary by state.

B. Psychiatric Management

1. Establish an alliance with the patient and family.

- Provide emotional support and guidance to patients and families, who are often frightened.
- Rely on the family and caregivers for information about the patient.
- Enlist the patient's family and caregivers to implement and monitor the treatment plan.
- Demonstrate compassion and concern for the patient's family and caregivers, since their attitudes and behaviors have a profound effect on the patient.

2. Educate the patient and family.

- Provide up-to-date information on the patient's illness.
- Review expected symptoms and course of illness.
- Describe available treatment options.
- Support realistic expectations.
- Facilitate education by providing written material, referral to the Alzheimer's Association, and referral to local social service agencies.

3. Advise the family about sources of care and support.

Potential sources include
- support groups,
- day care,
- respite care,
- assisted living facilities,
- nursing homes, and
- the Alzheimer's Association (www.alz.org).

4. Provide guidance on legal and financial issues.

- Encourage patient participation as indicated. Getting the patient involved relatively early in the course of the illness gives the patient a chance to provide input into current and future decisions.
- Plan with the patient and family for an orderly transfer of financial responsibility.
- Suggest that the patient execute critical documents such as wills, health care proxies, and durable power of attorney for medical and financial decisions. Alternatively, refer the patient and family to an expert in legal and financial planning.
- Help the patient and family plan for the cost of long-term care at home or in a nursing home or other facility. This should be discussed relatively early so that suitable preparations can be made.

5. Address special aspects of care for patients in nursing home settings.

Optimize the setting.
- Many patients with dementia eventually require nursing home placement. Approximately two-thirds of patients in long-term care have dementia.
- Structure facilities to meet the needs of patients with dementia.
- Carefully train staff.
- Provide an appropriate level of activity.
- Structure the living unit to contain wandering and minimize the risk of falls.
- There is no evidence that special care units are more effective than traditional units.

Minimize use of antipsychotic medications.
- Used appropriately, antipsychotics can be helpful in reducing agitation and psychosis and increasing safety for the patient, other residents, and staff.
- Overuse can lead to cognitive worsening, oversedation, falls, and tardive dyskinesia.
- Good clinical practice and federal regulations require careful consideration and documentation of indications for and alternatives to antipsychotic medications.
- Periodically consider decreasing the dose of antipsychotic medications or discontinuing them.
- Educate staff to limit use.

Minimize use of physical restraints.
- Use physical restraints only for patients who pose a significant risk of physical harm to themselves or others, and only while awaiting more definitive treatment.
- Address underlying causes of agitation promptly.
- Environmental changes may decrease the need for restraints by controlling wandering and minimizing the risk of falls.
- Carefully document indications for and alternatives to physical restraints.
- Observe legal and regulatory requirements.

C. General Treatment Principles

1. Development of a Treatment Plan

Assess the stage of illness and the nature and severity of problems.
Patients with dementia display a broad range of cognitive and functional impairments, behavioral disturbances, and mood symptoms. They require an individualized and multimodal treatment plan. Because dementia is often progressive, treatment must evolve to address emerging issues.

At each stage, be vigilant about expected symptoms.

Stage of Impairment		Likely Symptoms
Mild	Patient has difficulties limited to complex tasks such as balancing a checkbook.	• Depression • Awareness of and frustration with deficits
Moderate	Patient has difficulty completing simple household tasks.	• Depression • Development of psychotic symptoms such as paranoia
Severe	Patient requires assistance with basic activities of daily living such as personal hygiene.	• Psychosis • Agitation
Profound	Patient is terminal and totally dependent.	• Bedbound with significant motor deficits • Feeding difficulties • Incontinence

Help the patient and family plan for future symptoms.
• Prepare the patient and family emotionally.
• Help the patient and family arrange for the care likely to be required.
• Encourage legal and financial planning.

2. Psychosocial Treatments

In addition to the psychosocial interventions included in Psychiatric Management (section B, p. 17), a number of more specific interventions may help some patients with dementia. Although the goals of these treatments are nonspecific and research data are limited, clinical practice suggests that improvements in behavior, function, and mood may occur with the following interventions:

Behavior-oriented treatments
- These treatments try to identify the antecedents and consequences of problem behaviors and plan changes in the environment to minimize the behaviors and their consequences.
- These treatments are frequently effective in lessening or abolishing problem behaviors (e.g., aggression, screaming, incontinence).

Stimulation-oriented treatments
- These treatments include activities or recreational therapies (e.g., crafts, games, pets) and art therapies (e.g., music, dance, art).
- Clinical trials suggest that these treatments may be associated with modest improvements in cognition, function, and mood.
- Common sense supports use of these treatments as part of the humane care of patients with dementia.

Emotion-oriented treatments
- Reminiscence therapy stimulates memory and mood in the context of the patient's life history. Such therapy may be associated with modest short-lived gains in memory, behavior, and cognition.
- Other interventions include supportive psychotherapy, validation therapy (validates the patient's emotional ties to the past), sensory integration, and simulated presence therapy.
- Little or no evidence supports validation therapy, sensory integration, or simulated presence therapy.

2. Psychosocial Treatments (continued)

Cognition-oriented treatments
- Examples of cognition-oriented treatment include reality orientation, cognitive retraining, and skills training.
- These treatments may lead to slight transient improvements in a variety of domains, but reality orientation has been associated with frustration in some patients.

Treatments directed at caregivers
- Examples of treatment for caregivers include supportive psychotherapy, support groups offering education and emotional support, and respite care.
- These interventions are likely to be helpful to the caregiver and consequently may benefit patients as well.

3. Psychopharmacological Treatments

Start low and go slow.
Psychotropic medications should be used with caution. Elderly individuals tend to have decreased renal clearance and slowed hepatic metabolism, so lower starting dosages, smaller increases in dosage, and longer intervals between increments must be used.

Anticipate greater sensitivity to medication side effects.
The following medication side effects pose particular concerns in the elderly:
- Anticholinergic effects may lead to worsening cognitive impairment, confusion, and even delirium. (Coexisting cardiovascular disease, prostate or bladder disease, and other general medical conditions can be exacerbated by anticholinergic medications.)
- Orthostasis can lead to falls and associated injuries.
- Sedation may worsen cognitive functioning, predispose to falls, and in those with sleep apnea cause respiratory depression.
- Extrapyramidal symptoms may occur, especially in patients with Parkinson's disease.

Be alert to the impact of general medical conditions.
General medical conditions and the medications used to treat them may
- cause direct effects on the brain (e.g., stroke) and
- alter the binding, metabolism, and excretion of many medications.

Employ psychopharmacological treatments with care.
- Consider available alternatives to pharmacological intervention whenever possible.
- Delineate target symptoms carefully and discontinue ineffective treatments.
- Individualize dosing and choose the lowest effective dose for each patient.
- Be particularly careful when more than one agent is required.
- For some medications, periodic tapers or medication holidays may be beneficial.

D. Treatment of Specific Target Symptoms

1. Treatment of Cognitive and Functional Losses

Cholinesterase inhibitors
- Consideration of a trial with a cholinesterase inhibitor is warranted, given the lack of established alternatives and given that cholinesterase inhibitors yield modest improvement in some patients with mild to moderate cognitive impairment.
- Principal side effects are nausea, vomiting, increased gastrointestinal acid, and bradycardia.
- Donepezil is preferred over tacrine, which has similar modest efficacy but requires gradual dosage titration, q.i.d. dosing, and frequent monitoring (reversible elevations in liver enzyme levels occur in 30% of patients).

Vitamin E
- Vitamin E (2000 IU/day) may be used for patients with moderate Alzheimer's disease to delay disease progression.
- Although vitamin E has not been studied in patients with mild or severe disease, some physicians might consider it for patients in these stages as well, given its favorable side effect profile.
- Given its lack of medication interactions, vitamin E may be considered for use in combination with cholinesterase inhibitors.
- It should not be used, especially in high doses, in patients with vitamin K deficiency.

Selegiline
- Selegiline (5 mg b.i.d.) may be used for patients with moderate Alzheimer's disease to delay disease progression.
- Side effects include orthostatic hypotension, activation, and, because it is a selective monoamine oxidase B inhibitor, the potential for serious drug interactions (including hypertensive crisis). However, no tyramine-free diet or avoidance of sympathomimetic amines is needed.
- Vitamin E is often preferred over selegiline because it is equally efficacious in slowing decline, has a better side effect profile, and is less prone to medication interactions.
- However, a trial of selegiline should be considered, especially for patients who cannot take cholinesterase inhibitors, because limited evidence suggests it provides cognitive and functional improvement and limits decline. No benefits of combined treatment with vitamin E have been shown.

Hydergine (ergoloid mesylates)
- Hydergine is generally not recommended for patients with Alzheimer's disease because of questionable efficacy in numerous clinical trials.
- For patients with Alzheimer's disease for whom other options are inappropriate or unsuccessful, a trial may be appropriate.
- Somewhat more compelling evidence suggests it provides modest improvement in vascular dementia.

Other agents
- A number of other agents have been suggested as possible treatments for cognitive losses and are undergoing clinical trials.
- Data on ginkgo biloba are limited, results are variable, and preparations are not standardized and are of unknown quality.
- Estrogen, nonsteroidal anti-inflammatory agents, and anti-inflammatory COX-2 inhibitors cannot be recommended because there is no evidence of efficacy and adverse effects may be significant.
- For some patients, formal clinical trials of these or other experimental agents may be an appropriate option.

2. Treatment of Psychosis and Agitation

Evaluation and initial intervention
- Psychosis and agitation are common in dementia.
- Review the safety of the patient and others and intervene as necessary.
- Perform a careful medical evaluation. Agitation can result from an occult general medical problem, untreated or undertreated pain, depression, sleep loss, or delirium. The agitation will often resolve with treatment of the underlying condition.
- Assess the patient's overall situation: agitation can also result from physical discomfort, such as hunger or sleep deprivation; an interpersonal issue, such as a change in living situation; or an emotional difficulty, such as frustration, boredom, or loneliness. Attending to unmet needs, providing reassurance, or redirecting activities may resolve the problem.
- If symptoms remain, and if they do not cause danger to the patient or caregivers or undue distress to the patient, treat with reassurance and distraction.
- For agitation, behavioral interventions may be helpful.
- Treat psychosis or agitation pharmacologically when such behavior is dangerous or upsetting.
- Educate caregivers.

Benzodiazepines
- Benzodiazepines should not be used on a regular basis except for patients with prominent anxiety.
- Benzodiazepines may also be used as needed for patients with infrequent episodes of agitation who require sedation or for a procedure such as a tooth extraction.
- In treating behavioral symptoms, benzodiazepines work better than placebo, but not as well as antipsychotics.
- Side effects include sedation, increased risk of falls, and worsening cognition.
- Lorazepam and oxazepam are probably the best choices among the benzodiazepines. They have no active metabolites and do not depend on the liver for their metabolism.

Anticonvulsants
- Consider carbamazepine and divalproex sodium for the treatment of agitation.
- Both agents have modest support in clinical trials.
- Both agents can lead to confusion and ataxia and carry a slight risk of blood dyscrasias.

Other agents
- The sedating antidepressant trazodone and the atypical anxiolytic agent buspirone may both be considered for the treatment of agitation, based primarily on case reports and small clinical trials.
- Lithium and beta-blockers are not recommended. There is little evidence for efficacy, and potential side effects are serious.

3. Treatment of Depression

Assess safety, including potential for suicide and adequacy of nutrition.

Treat all patients with depressed mood.
- Depression is common in dementia.
- Assess all patients for suicide potential.
- Depressed mood may respond to improvements in living situation or to stimulation-oriented treatments. If not, patients with depressive symptoms should be treated with antidepressant medications even if their mood disturbance does not meet criteria for major depressive disorder.

3. Treatment of Depression *(continued)*

Select an agent.
- Formal evaluation of antidepressant efficacy is limited in patients with dementia, but there is considerable clinical evidence of efficacy. Management of depression in individuals with dementia is generally similar to that in elderly individuals without dementia.
- The choice of agent is based on side effect profile.
- Selective serotonin reuptake inhibitors (SSRIs) will often be the first choice because of their favorable side effect profiles.
- Other agents such as bupropion, venlafaxine, and tricyclic antidepressants may be appropriate for some patients.
- Agents with significant anticholinergic effects (e.g., amitriptyline, imipramine) should be avoided.
- Monoamine oxidase inhibitors should be used only when other agents have failed.

Consider electroconvulsive therapy.
- Clinical experience suggests that electroconvulsive therapy is effective when medications fail.
- Twice- rather than thrice-weekly and unilateral rather than bilateral treatments may decrease the risk of delirium and memory loss associated with this modality.

4. Treatment of Sleep Disturbances

Attempt behavioral interventions first.
- Before instituting pharmacological treatment, recommend appropriate sleep hygiene measures (e.g., a predictable and calming bedtime routine, regulation of light and noise).
- If the treatment setting provides adequate supervision, permitting daytime sleep and nocturnal awakening may provide an alternative to pharmacological intervention.

Select sedating medications for other indications.
If the patient has a sleep disturbance and also requires medication for another indication (e.g., depression, psychosis, agitation), an agent with sedating properties (e.g., trazodone or nortriptyline for depression) should be selected, if possible, and administered at bedtime.

Consider pharmacological options for sleep.
• Consider zolpidem and trazodone.
• Use benzodiazepines and chloral hydrate only briefly. Long-term use is not recommended because of the risk of tolerance, rebound insomnia, and disinhibition.
• Avoid triazolam (because of its association with amnesia) and diphenhydramine (because of its anticholinergic properties).
• Sleep apnea is relatively common in the elderly and is a contraindication to the use of benzodiazepines or other agents that suppress respiratory drive.

TREATING HIV/AIDS
A Quick Reference Guide

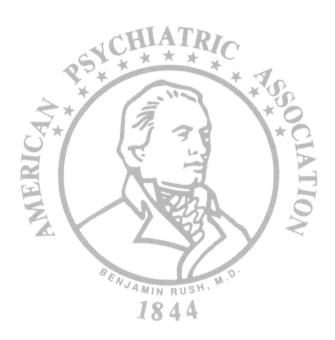

Based on *Practice Guideline for the Treatment of Patients With HIV/AIDS,*
originally published in November 2000. A guideline watch, summarizing significant
developments in the scientific literature since publication of this guideline, may be available
in the Psychiatric Practice section of the APA web site at www.psych.org.

OUTLINE

A. General Information on HIV/AIDS

1. Epidemiology

- Current U.S. information is available at www.cdc.gov/hiv/dhap.htm.
- Since 1995, there has been a large decline in death rates because of antiretroviral therapy.
- The overall prevalence of HIV/AIDS has increased because of decline in death rates plus the steady rate of new HIV infection; prevention of infection remains a high priority.

2. Transmission of HIV

Routes of transmission
- *Sexual:* Unprotected intercourse is the most common route of transmission, irrespective of gender or sexual orientation.
- *Injection drug use:* Sharing unsterilized injection equipment is a very efficient means of transmitting HIV.
- *Perinatal:* Infection from mother to infant can occur during gestation, delivery, or breast-feeding.
- *Blood transfusion:* In the U.S., screening blood for HIV has reduced the risk by transfusion to almost zero.

Cofactors that enhance transmission
- *Physical:* The presence of sexually transmitted diseases may cause genital lesions or genital/mucous membrane bleeding during sexual activity.
- *Behavioral:* Substance use lowers sexual inhibitions, impairs judgment, and increases impulsivity.

3. Pathogenesis of HIV

- During the acute phase, 50% to 90% of people experience a flulike syndrome within 3 to 6 weeks of infection.
- The clinically asymptomatic phase may last for many years. The host seroconverts. The immune system may appear to control infection, but chronic viral replication persists.
- AIDS is defined by conditions indicating significant immuno-suppression (e.g., opportunistic infections) or other conditions (dementia, wasting). For criteria, see Appendix A (p. 50) in this guide and Table 4 of APA's *Practice Guideline for the Treatment of Patients With HIV/AIDS.*

4. Antiretroviral Treatment

- For guidelines on the use of antiretroviral agents, go to www.aidsinfo.nih.gov.
- The goal of antiretroviral treatment is to reduce viral load to undetectable levels and maintain this without interruption.
- Lack of clinical response may be due to problems with adherence, suboptimal antiretroviral treatment potency, or genetic mutation of strains.
- Adverse effects of antiretroviral treatment include lipodystrophy (fat redistribution syndromes), hyperlipidemia, nephrotoxicity, bone marrow suppression, neuropathy, nausea, diarrhea, sleep disturbances, rash, and elevation of glucose levels, possibly causing diabetes mellitus.
- Combined cost for antiretroviral agents in multidrug regimens is very expensive.
- Adherence is of utmost concern with antiretroviral treatment. Even minor deviations from the prescribed regimen can result in viral resistance and permanent loss of efficacy. Studies of antiretroviral treatment continue to indicate that near-perfect adherence is needed to adequately repress viral replication.

B. Management of Individuals at High Risk

1. Assessment

Obtain risk history.
- Risk history should be considered in every psychiatric evaluation to identify individuals at high risk.
- An ongoing appraisal of risk is sometimes needed (e.g., during acute episodes of psychiatric illness, stressful or traumatic life events, and initiation of sexual activity in adolescents).
- Sexual history should be assessed with nonjudgmental attitude (see Table 2 of APA's *Practice Guideline for the Treatment of Patients With HIV/AIDS* for risks associated with specific behaviors).
- See Table 12 of APA's *Practice Guideline for the Treatment of Patients With HIV/AIDS* for risk assessment questions.

Conform to the vocabulary and cultural beliefs of the patient.
See www.drugabuse.gov for a current list of drug terminology.

2. HIV Antibody Testing

Identify infection early.
- Early identification of HIV infection is important so that newly infected persons can be medically monitored and promptly receive antiretroviral treatment as appropriate.
- Risks of testing include worries, fears, and stigma associated with a diagnosis of HIV/AIDS.

2. HIV Antibody Testing (continued)

Provide pre- and posttest counseling.
- Explain the HIV test, including risks and benefits.
- Discuss the confidentiality of results.
- Review risk behaviors and present risk reduction strategies.
- Discuss plans for dealing with a positive or negative result.

Centers for Disease Control and Prevention (CDC) guidelines for counseling are available at www.cdc.gov/hiv/pubs.htm.

Discuss with the patient issues surrounding disclosure of status to family, friends, or employers.

The American College of Obstetricians and Gynecologists recommends that an HIV antibody test be offered during annual examinations to all women seeking preconception care.

3. Risk Reduction Strategies

Provide education about behaviors that place patients at risk for HIV infection.

Manage risk behaviors.
- Active discussions foster changes in behavior.
- Ongoing discussions about motivation and skills are needed to ensure consistent changes.
- Problems or disorders that may promote risky behavior include impulse control disorders, untreated depression, hypersexuality associated with mania, psychotic disorders, mental disorders due to a general medical condition, binge alcohol or drug use, and personality disorders.
- Extended counseling and case management should be provided for continuing management of risk behaviors.

Implement specific risk reduction programs (e.g., needle-exchange programs, skills training groups).

Help the patient develop skills to discuss and negotiate safer sex with partners (e.g., practice communication skills through role-play).

Evaluate the patient's access to condoms and skills to use them. See Table 13 of APA's *Practice Guideline for the Treatment of Patients With HIV/AIDS* for guidelines on condom use.

4. Postexposure Prophylaxis

- Postexposure prophylaxis (PEP) may prevent initial cellular infection and local propagation of HIV.
- PEP is currently recommended for known occupational exposure, especially percutaneous or mucous membrane exposure to blood or other bodily fluids. Its value in other exposure situations (e.g., known sexual exposure) is being studied.
- Rapid assessment is essential. A multiple-drug regimen must begin as soon as 1 to 2 hours and no later than 24 to 36 hours after exposure. The regimen must continue for at least 4 weeks.

Additional information is available through the National Clinicians' Postexposure Prophylaxis Hotline (888-448-4911) and web site (www.ucsf.edu/hivcntr).

5. Special Populations of Patients

Patients with severe mental disorders
- HIV infection may be associated with health risks caused by poor access to health care or by decreased capacity for self-care.
- Risk reduction programs tailored to the needs of this special population have been shown to reduce the risk of HIV infection.

Patients with substance use disorders
- For patients injecting drugs, risk reduction strategies include methadone or LAAM maintenance treatment, needle-use education and bleach distribution, drug rehabilitation programs, safer-sex education, legal clean-needle purchase, and needle-exchange programs.
- For noninjection drugs and alcohol, treatment may reduce risk exposure secondary to disinhibition or cognitive impairment.

Victims of sexual abuse/crimes
- Ask about specific behaviors that are associated with the risk of HIV transmission.
- Determine whether a psychiatric disorder is present and whether treatment is indicated.
- Consider PEP in cases of sexual assault.

C. Psychiatric Management of Individuals With HIV/AIDS

1. Assessment

Obtain risk history; determine HIV status.

Conduct a comprehensive diagnostic evaluation.
Because of the stress associated with HIV diagnosis, special attention should be paid to assessing suicidal ideation, self-destructive behavior, and extreme anger.

Assess possible medical causes of new-onset symptoms and initiate specific treatment interventions.

Understand psychodynamic issues.

Include HIV risk assessment and prevention in the treatment plan for every patient with severe mental illness and/or an alcohol or substance use disorder.

2. Management Principles

Establish and maintain a therapeutic alliance.
- Determine the patient's understanding of stage of illness and evaluate coping mechanisms.
- Explore cultural/ethnic beliefs regarding psychiatric and HIV illness and conform to the language of the patient.
- Review issues of confidentiality. The patient should be asked to consider the psychiatrist's role in assisting in the process of disclosure of HIV status to appropriate persons.
- Be aware of transference and countertransference feelings, including personal attitudes about HIV infection and how the patient acquired it.

2. Management Principles *(continued)*

Coordinate care with other mental health and medical providers.
• It is essential to collaborate with other physicians practicing in infectious disease, primary care, and other disciplines to keep up to date—for example, through discussions of drug interactions and close monitoring and workup of unexplained or psychiatric symptoms.
• Patients need to agree to the exchange of specific information with other care providers.

Diagnose and treat all associated psychiatric disorders.
• Actively monitor for substance abuse, because it is often associated with risk behaviors.
• Do not assume that patients who have relatively good immune functioning have no risk for CNS HIV disorders.
• Note that psychotherapeutic management of patients with HIV infection is similar to that of other patients.

Facilitate adherence to overall treatment plan.
• See Appendix B (p. 51) in this guide for strategies to increase adherence.
• Poor adherence to antiretroviral medications results in development of viral resistance.
• Comorbid psychiatric disorders (e.g., substance abuse or depression) can adversely affect adherence; adherence to both psychotropic and HIV medications is important.
• Psychoeducational approaches can reinforce the importance of adherence, encourage the patient to seek appropriate help from others, and identify barriers to adherence.
• Intensive psychodynamic psychotherapy may be helpful if the patient is still unable to modify behavior after educational approaches.
• Outreach efforts with public health nurses and services can provide adherence assistance for hard-to-reach patients.

Provide risk reduction strategies to minimize the spread of HIV.
- Risk reduction is an ongoing treatment priority.
- Risk assessment should be repeated when there are changes in the clinical status or social situation.
- Patients on high-dose antiretroviral medications should be advised that they remain contagious.

Help the patient maximize psychological and social/adaptive functioning.
- Assess social supports.
- Use appropriate community-based services.
- Encourage the patient to resolve legal and financial concerns, providing assistance when necessary.
- Assist with significant intrapersonal, interpersonal, and social stresses.

Explore the role of religion and spirituality in the patient's care.

Prepare the patient for issues of disability, dying, and death.
- Evaluate the need for work or school accommodations in line with the Americans With Disabilities Act.
- Assist the patient in drawing up a living will to guide end-of-life decisions.

Advise significant others, including family, about sources of care and support.
- Refer to support groups.
- Encourage participation in HIV/AIDS advocacy organizations.
- Consider referral of significant others and family for psychiatric evaluation and treatment, including individual or family therapy.

D. Management of HIV-Related Neuropsychiatric Symptoms

1. Assessment
a. Differential Diagnosis

Delirium
- Delirium should be considered before other diagnoses.
- Delirium is common in HIV infection.
- Most common causes are iatrogenic and psychoactive-substance–induced toxicity, infection, neoplasms, metabolic disturbances, some antiretroviral medications (e.g., zidovudine at high doses).

Other HIV-associated cognitive dysfunction

HIV-associated dementia (HAD)
- Subcortical dementia
- Clinical triad of progressive cognitive decline, motor dysfunction, and behavioral abnormalities
- Common symptoms: psychomotor slowing, decreased speed of information processing, impaired verbal memory and learning efficiency, impairment in executive functioning

HIV-associated minor cognitive motor disorder (MCMD)
- Less severe than HAD
- Important to diagnose and treat because it involves dysfunction rather than cell death
- May affect spinal column (e.g., vascular myelopathy of dorsolateral columns) and/or peripheral nerves (e.g., painful sensory neuropathy)

(continued)

HIV-associated progressive encephalopathy (PE) or HIV encephalopathy in children (terms used instead of "dementia caused by HIV")
- Condition is characterized by a triad of symptoms: impaired brain growth, progressive motor dysfunction, and loss or plateau of developmental milestones.
- Markers of immunological functioning (e.g., CD4 count) do not correlate with degree of neurocognitive impairment.
- Some cognitive and language delays (e.g., receptive and expressive language and visual-motor deficits) are present even when the patient appears asymptomatic.
- Condition should be distinguished from mental retardation secondary to other causes, such as maternal drug addiction and prematurity, which can be determined only by longitudinal assessment.

Mental disorders caused by general medical conditions affecting the CNS
Patient may present with psychiatric symptoms or syndromes such as psychosis or mood disorder (see Appendix C, p. 52, in this guide).

Medication-induced mental disorders
Medications commonly used to treat conditions associated with HIV infection may have psychiatric symptoms as side effects (see Appendix D, p. 53, in this guide).

1. Assessment
b. Workup of Acute Changes in Mental Status

Rule out treatable and reversible medical causes—especially if CD4 counts drop or viral load rises. Note that acute changes in mental status may *not* correlate with changes in CD4 counts or viral load and may be due to other causes.

1. Assessment
b. Workup of Acute Changes in Mental Status (continued)

Workup for patients with or at high risk for HIV infection who present with acute onset with no previous psychiatric history:
- Complete medical evaluation, including physical/neurological examination (see Appendix C, p. 52, in this guide for CNS manifestations of HIV infection)
  - Focal deficits may indicate a space-occupying lesion.
  - Sensory changes may indicate peripheral neuropathy.
  - Ataxia or changes in gait may indicate myelopathy.
- Oxygen saturation of blood and, in patients with pneumonia, arterial blood gas
- Laboratory analyses
  - Complete blood count (CBC) with differential
  - Serum chemistries
  - VDRL, fluorescent treponemal antibody
  - Vitamin B_{12}, folate levels
  - CD4 count and viral load
  - Toxicology screen
- Brain imaging studies to rule out space-occupying lesion
- Comprehensive assessment to rule out infectious processes; consider lumbar puncture
- Neuropsychological testing (e.g., AIDS Dementia Rating Scale, Finger Tapping Test, Trail Making Test)

1. Assessment
c. Evaluation of Cognitive Symptoms

- A comprehensive psychiatric assessment, formulation of a differential diagnosis, and possible medical workup are required.
- Differentiate subcortical from cortical involvement: early cognitive changes differ from symptoms associated with cortical dementia; more commonly presents with psychomotor slowing, short-term memory dysfunction, or attention deficits rather than deficits in language or visual recognition.   *(continued)*

- Mini-Mental State Exam (MMSE) is not sensitive in picking up early HIV-associated cognitive-motor symptoms (see Table 14 of APA's *Practice Guideline for the Treatment of Patients With HIV/AIDS* for a list of sensitive screening examinations).
- Patient self-assessment is not reliable.
- Baseline screening examination should be done on every patient with HIV.
- Cognitive screening examinations should be readministered on a regular basis.
- Once cognitive dysfunction is identified, formal neuropsychological testing is helpful to fully document dysfunction and identify areas of relative strength when there is evidence of impairment.
- Once the symptoms are identified, the practitioner should collaborate with other clinicians regarding further medical care.

2. Treatment

Delirium

- Treat delirium per APA's *Practice Guideline for the Treatment of Patients With Delirium* (also see "Treating Delirium: A Quick Reference Guide," p. 1). Intervention should correct underlying causes (see Appendix E, p. 54, in this guide for a list of etiologies).

Dementia

- Use potent antiretroviral therapy to target the underlying HIV infection.
- Use psychotropic medication for comorbid conditions such as depression.
- Consider antipsychotic or stimulant agents for symptomatic management of HIV-associated dementia (e.g., agitation or fatigue).
- Consider psychotherapy for mild to moderate dementia to help patients understand, mourn, and adapt to this new impairment of functioning.

E. Management of Other Disorders

1. General Treatment Guidelines

➤ **Provide psychotherapy.**
Psychotherapeutic management of patients with HIV infection should follow the same general principles used with other patients.

➤ **Provide pharmacotherapy.**

For all HIV-infected patients:
- Follow principles similar to those for geriatric patients or patients with comorbid medical illnesses.
- Be aware that some medications for HIV can potently inhibit or induce the cytochrome P450 (CYP450) system (see Appendix F, p. 55, in this guide).
- Judiciously use psychotropics that share metabolic pathways.

Particularly for patients with symptomatic HIV disease:
- Use lower starting doses and slower titration.
- Provide the least complicated dosing schedules possible.
- Focus on drug side effect profiles to avoid unnecessary adverse effects (e.g., anticholinergic effects from tricyclic antidepressants, leukopenia from carbamazepine).
- Maintain awareness of drug metabolism/clearance pathways and possible end-organ effects to minimize drug-drug interactions.
- Collaborate with primary HIV provider to ensure that all medications prescribed are compatible.

2. Psychiatric Disorders

Mood disorders
- Management of mood disorders is similar to that for other mood disorders with medical comorbidity.
- Fatigue and insomnia may be symptomatic of the mood disorder, especially in medically asymptomatic patients.
- The overall medical status of the patient should be assessed to take into account possible effects of concurrent illness or side effects of medication.
- Choice (and dosage) of antidepressant or mood-stabilizing agent may be influenced by the antiretroviral regimen.

Substance use disorders
- Substance use disorders should be treated (e.g., with a drug rehabilitation program) to reduce risk behavior in order to prevent further infection of others.
- During treatment of opiate dependence with methadone or LAAM, doses may need to be increased or decreased in accordance with the use of specific antiretroviral agents.

Anxiety disorders
- Psychotherapeutic approaches to situational anxiety can help patients work through intense affects.
- Standard pharmacological treatments for anxiety disorders should be used with caution (e.g., many benzodiazepines should be used very cautiously when patients are taking protease inhibitors, particularly ritonavir, because benzodiazepine blood levels may be greatly elevated).

2. Psychiatric Disorders (continued)

Psychotic disorders
- Psychotic symptomatology may arise from opportunistic infections, mania, HIV-associated dementia, or delirium.
- Evaluation of new-onset psychosis requires a careful medical/neurological workup.
- Practitioners should beware of drug-drug interactions and overlapping toxicities (e.g., ritonavir may elevate levels of clozapine; clozapine and zidovudine both cause bone marrow suppression).
- Atypical neuroleptics are first-line treatments in late-stage HIV infection because of lower incidence of extrapyramidal side effects.
- Lower doses of atypical antipsychotics tend to be sufficient.

Adjustment disorders
- Various forms of psychotherapy may be indicated to prevent progression to a more severe psychiatric disturbance.

Sleep disorders
- May be secondary to a psychiatric disorder such as depression.
- May be a manifestation of HIV infection in the brain.
- May be secondary to complications of HIV infection (e.g., pain); medical intervention may improve sleep.
- Efavirenz (an antiretroviral) is associated with a high incidence of vivid dreams and nightmares.

Disorders of infancy, childhood, and adolescence
- Psychiatric disorders are common among infected youth, with rates of about 30% for mood disorders and 25% for attention-deficit/hyperactivity disorder.
- Psychotherapy may be of particular help for adolescents who are struggling with emerging sexuality.
- Substance abuse in adolescents is frequent and likely to involve multiple drugs.
- Issues of risk behavior and autonomy have implications for HIV prevention, adherence to treatment, and effective coping with chronic illness.

3. HIV-Associated Syndromes With Psychiatric Implications

- Somatic symptoms at the interface of medical and psychiatric disorders include fatigue, weight loss, pain, and sexual dysfunction. Psychiatrists can integrate treatment approaches and promote interdisciplinary and interspecialty dialogue; they should avoid all-or-nothing, mind-or-body approaches.
- Wasting syndrome generally occurs in patients with more advanced HIV illness and can be related to a number of physiological disturbances such as progressive HIV disease, hypogonadism, and gastrointestinal malabsorption.
- Chronic fatigue is frequently associated with depressed mood and physical disability.
- Common painful symptoms include headaches, herpetic lesions, peripheral neuropathy, back pain, throat pain, arthralgias, and muscle and abdominal pain.
- Sexual dysfunction has been reported to occur in both men and women with HIV infection. In both men and women, hypogonadism can be treated with testosterone replacement with physiological dosing.

APPENDIX A. 1993 Revised Classification System for HIV Infection and Expanded AIDS Surveillance Case Definition for AIDS Among Adolescents and Adults

	Clinical Categories		
	A	B	C
T cell count (cells/μL)	Acute (primary) HIV or persistent generalized lymphadenopathy; patient is asymptomatic	Patient is symptomatic, but condition does not meet criteria for category A or C	Patient has an AIDS indicator condition[a]
≥500	A1	B1	C1
200–499	A2	B2	C2
<200[a]	A3	B3	C3

[a]As of Jan. 1, 1993, persons with AIDS indicator conditions (categories C1–C3) as well as those with T lymphocyte counts less than 200/μL (category A3 or B3) were categorized as AIDS cases in the United States and its territories.

Source. From Centers for Disease Control and Prevention: "1993 Revised Classification System for HIV Infection and Expanded Surveillance Case Definition for AIDS Among Adolescents and Adults." MMWR 41(RR-17):1–19, 1992.

APPENDIX B. Interventions to Increase Patient Adherence to Antiretroviral Regimens

Prepare patients.
- Discuss use of medications before prescribing.
- Outline pros and cons of therapy.
- Acknowledge commitment required, consequences of nonadherence, and benefits of therapy.

Provide written instructions.
- Inform patients of expectations, including side effects.
- Provide information about whom patients should call if significant side effects occur.
- Schedule a follow-up appointment soon after initiating therapy.

Review importance of therapy.
- Inform patients that they must continue to take all medications.
- Review the effects of stopping one medication.
- Outline procedure for obtaining refills.

Recognize patient lifestyle and preferences.
- Twice-daily dosing benefits may outweigh initial side effects; ritonavir may be preferred.
- Consider whether patients prefer tolerability over convenience; nelfinavir or indinavir may be preferred.
- Discuss midday dosing.
- Recommend medication timers or calendar.
- Help patients plan for away-from-home dosing.
- Simplify regimens.
- If possible, prioritize or eliminate medications when patients are overwhelmed.

Look for and address nonadherence.
- Consider regimens that minimize cross-resistance.
- Use regimens that leave options for future effective antiretroviral therapy.
- Inquire about adherence.
- Inquire about medication-taking behavior at each visit.
- Anticipate relapses in adherence, even after long-term use of medication.

APPENDIX C. CNS Manifestations of HIV-1 Infection

Type of Manifestation	Condition
Acute HIV-1 infection	• Viral meningitis • Encephalitis • Ascending polyneuropathy
Opportunistic infections (late HIV-1 infection)	• Toxoplasma cerebritis • Cryptococcal meningitis • Progressive multifocal leukoencephalopathy • Neurosyphilis • *Mycobacterium tuberculosis* meningitis • Cytomegalovirus encephalitis • Herpes simplex encephalitis
Neoplastic disease (late HIV-1 infection)	• CNS lymphoma • Kaposi's sarcoma
Other manifestations	• HIV-associated cognitive dysfunctions (see section D.1.a, p. 42, in this guide)

APPENDIX D. Neuropsychiatric Side Effects of Selected Medications Used in HIV Disease

Drug	Target Illness	Side Effects
Acyclovir	Herpes encephalitis	• Visual hallucinations, depersonalization, tearfulness, confusion, hyperesthesia, hyperacusis, thought insertion, insomnia
Amphotericin B	Cryptococcosis	• Delirium, peripheral neuropathy, diplopia
β-Lactam antibiotics	Infections	• Confusion, paranoia, hallucinations, mania, coma
Co-trimoxazole	*Pneumocystis carinii* pneumonia	• Depression, loss of appetite, insomnia, apathy
Cycloserine	Tuberculosis	• Psychosis, somnolence, depression, confusion, tremor, vertigo, paresis, seizures, dysarthria
Didanosine	HIV	• Nervousness, anxiety, confusion, seizures, insomnia, peripheral neuropathy
Efavirenz	HIV	• Nightmares, depression, confusion
Foscarnet	Cytomegalovirus	• Paresthesias, seizures, headache, irritability, hallucinations, confusion
Interferon-α	Kaposi's sarcoma	• Depression, weakness, headache, myalgias, confusion
Isoniazid	Tuberculosis	• Depression, agitation, hallucinations, paranoia, impaired memory, anxiety
Lamivudine	HIV	• Insomnia, mania
Methotrexate	Lymphoma	• Encephalopathy (at high dose)
Pentamidine	*Pneumocystis carinii* pneumonia	• Confusion, anxiety, lability, hallucinations
Procarbazine	Lymphoma	• Mania, loss of appetite, insomnia, nightmares, confusion, malaise
Quinolones	Infection	• Psychosis, delirium, seizures, anxiety, insomnia, depression
Stavudine	HIV	• Headache, asthenia, malaise, confusion, depression, seizures, excitability, anxiety, mania, early morning awakening, insomnia
Sulfonamides	Infection	• Psychosis, delirium, confusion, depression, hallucinations
Thiabendazole	Strongyloidiasis	• Hallucinations, olfactory disturbance
Vinblastine	Kaposi's sarcoma	• Depression, loss of appetite, headache
Vincristine	Kaposi's sarcoma	• Hallucinations, headache, ataxia, sensory loss
Zalcitabine	HIV	• Headache, confusion, impaired concentration, somnolence, asthenia, depression, seizures, peripheral neuropathy
Zidovudine	HIV	• Headache, malaise, asthenia, insomnia, unusually vivid dreams, restlessness, severe agitation, mania, auditory hallucinations, confusion

Source. Adapted from Grant I, Atkinson JH Jr: "Neuropsychiatric Aspects of HIV Infection and AIDS," in *Kaplan and Sadock's Comprehensive Textbook of Psychiatry.* Edited by Sadock BJ, Sadock VA. Philadelphia, PA, Lippincott Williams & Wilkins, 1999, pp. 308–336.

APPENDIX E. Etiologies of Delirium in Patients With HIV/AIDS

Intracranial
- Seizures
- Infections
- Cryptococcal meningitis
- Encephalitis due to HIV, herpes, cytomegalovirus
- Progressive multifocal leukoencephalopathy
- Mass lesions
- Lymphoma
- Toxoplasmosis

Extracranial
- Medications and other drugs (not exhaustive)
  - Amphotericin B
  - Acyclovir
  - Ganciclovir
  - Ethambutol
  - Trimethoprim/sulfamethoxazole
  - Pentamidine
  - Foscarnet
  - Ketoconazole
  - Sedative-hypnotics
  - Cycloserine
  - Opiate analgesics
  - Isoniazid
  - Rifampin
  - Zidovudine or didanosine
  - Vincristine
  - Dapsone
- Drug or alcohol withdrawal
- Infection/sepsis
- Endocrine dysfunction/metabolic abnormality
  - Hypoglycemia due to pentamidine, protease inhibitors
  - Hypoxia due to pneumonia
- Nonendocrine organ dysfunction
  - Renal failure due to HIV nephropathy or medication toxicity
  - Liver failure due to comorbid hepatitis and medication toxicity
- Nutritional deficiencies
  - Wasting syndrome
  - Failure to replace trace elements or vitamins in total parenteral nutrition

Source. Adapted from Bialer PA, Wallack JJ, McDaniel JS: "Human Immunodeficiency Virus and AIDS," in *Psychiatric Care of the Medical Patient.* Edited by Stoudemire A, Fogel BS, Greenberg DB. New York, Oxford University Press, 2000, pp. 871–888.

APPENDIX F. Antiretroviral Medications and Cytochrome P450 Inhibition or Induction

Class/Drug Name	Predominant Effects on CYP450 Enzymes	
	Inhibition	Induction
Protease inhibitors[a]		
Amprenavir	3A4	[b]
Indinavir	3A4	[b]
Lopinavir[c]	3A4	[b]
Nelfinavir	3A4, 2C19, 2D6	[b]
Ritonavir[c]	3A4, 2C9, 2D6	[b]
Saquinavir	3A4	[b]
Nonnucleoside reverse transcriptase inhibitors		
Delavirdine	3A4	[b]
Efavirenz	3A4	3A4, 2B6
Nevirapine	[b]	3A4, 2B6
Nucleoside analogue reverse transcriptase inhibitors		
Abacavir	[b]	[b]
Didanosine (formerly dideoxyinosine [ddl])	[b]	[b]
Lamivudine (formerly 3TC)[c]	[b]	[b]
Stavudine (formerly d4T)	[b]	[b]
Zalcitabine (formerly 2′3′-dideoxycytidine [ddC])	[b]	[b]
Zidovudine (formerly azidothymidine [AZT])[c]	[b]	[b]
Nucleotide analogues		
Tenofovir	[b]	[b]

[a]Relative rank ordering of CYP3A4 inhibition for protease inhibitors is ritonavir >> indinavir, nelfinavir, amprenavir > saquinavir.
[b]No clinically significant effect.
[c]Lamivudine-zidovudine and lopinavir-ritonavir are available as combination preparations.

TREATING
SCHIZOPHRENIA
A Quick Reference Guide

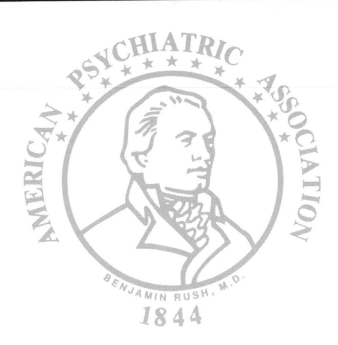

Based on *Practice Guideline for the Treatment of Patients With Schizophrenia*, Second Edition, originally published in February 2004. A guideline watch, summarizing significant developments in the scientific literature since publication of this guideline, may be available in the Psychiatric Practice section of the APA web site at www.psych.org.

OUTLINE

A. Psychiatric Management

1. Assess symptoms and establish a diagnosis.

→ Establish an accurate diagnosis, considering other psychotic disorders in the differential diagnosis because of the major implications for short- and long-term treatment planning. If a definitive diagnosis cannot be made but the patient appears prodromally symptomatic and at risk for psychosis, reevaluate the patient frequently.

→ Reevaluate the patient's diagnosis and update the treatment plan as new information about the patient and his or her symptoms becomes available.

→ Identify the targets of each treatment, use outcome measures that gauge the effect of treatment, and have realistic expectations about the degrees of improvement that constitute successful treatment.

→ Consider the use of objective, quantitative rating scales to monitor clinical status (e.g., Abnormal Involuntary Movement Scale [AIMS], Structured Clinical Interview for DSM-IV Axis I Disorders [SCID], Brief Psychiatric Rating Scale [BPRS], Positive and Negative Syndrome Scale [PANSS]).

2. Formulate and implement a treatment plan.

→ Select specific type(s) of treatment and the treatment setting. (This process is iterative and should evolve over the course of the patient's association with the clinician.)

3. Develop a therapeutic alliance and promote treatment adherence.

Identify the patient's goals and aspirations and relate these to treatment outcomes to increase treatment adherence.

Assess factors contributing to incomplete treatment adherence and implement clinical interventions (e.g., motivational interviewing) to address them. Factors contributing to incomplete treatment adherence include

- patient's lack of insight about presence of illness or need to take medication,
- patient's perceptions about lack of treatment benefits (e.g., inadequate symptom relief) and risks (e.g., unpleasant side effects, discrimination associated with being in treatment),
- cognitive impairment,
- breakdown of the therapeutic alliance,
- practical barriers such as financial concerns or lack of transportation,
- cultural beliefs, and
- lack of family or other social support.

Consider assertive outreach (including telephone calls and home visits) for patients who consistently do not appear for appointments or are nonadherent in other ways.

4. Provide patient and family education and therapies.

Work with patients to recognize early symptoms of relapse in order to prevent full-blown illness exacerbations.

Educate the family about the nature of the illness and coping strategies to diminish relapses and improve quality of life for patients.

5. Treat comorbid conditions, especially major depression, substance use disorders, and posttraumatic stress disorder.

6. Attend to the patient's social circumstances and functioning.

Work with team members, the patient, and the family to ensure that services are coordinated and that referrals for additional services are made when appropriate.

7. Integrate treatments from multiple clinicians.

8. Carefully document the treatment, since patients may have different practitioners over their course of illness.

B. Acute Phase

Goals of treatment
- Prevent harm.
- Control disturbed behavior.
- Reduce the severity of psychosis and associated symptoms (e.g., agitation, aggression, negative symptoms, affective symptoms).
- Determine and address the factors that led to the occurrence of the acute episode.
- Effect a rapid return to the best level of functioning.
- Develop an alliance with the patient and family.
- Formulate short- and long-term treatment plans.
- Connect the patient with appropriate aftercare in the community.

1. Assessment in the Acute Phase

Goals of acute phase assessment
- Evaluate the reason for the recurrence or exacerbation of symptoms (e.g., medication nonadherence).
- Determine or verify the patient's diagnosis.
- Identify any comorbid psychiatric or medical conditions, including substance use disorders.
- Evaluate general medical health.
- Identify the patient's strengths and limitations.
- Engage the patient in a therapeutic alliance.

Undertake a thorough initial workup, including complete psychiatric and general medical histories and physical and mental status examinations.

Routinely interview family members or other individuals knowledgeable about the patient, unless the patient refuses to grant permission.

In emergency circumstances (e.g., safety risk), it may be necessary and permissible to speak with others without the patient's consent.

Conduct laboratory tests, including a complete blood count (CBC); measurements of blood electrolytes and glucose; tests of liver, renal, and thyroid function; a syphilis test; and, when indicated, a urine or serum toxicology screen, hepatitis C test, and determination of HIV status.

Consider use of a computed tomography (CT) or magnetic resonance imaging (MRI) scan (MRI is preferred) for patients with a new onset of psychosis or with an atypical clinical presentation, because findings (e.g., ventricular enlargement, diminished cortical volume) may enhance confidence in the diagnosis and provide information relevant to treatment planning and prognosis.

Assess risk factors for suicide (such as prior attempts, depressed mood, suicidal ideation, presence of command hallucinations, hopelessness, anxiety, extrapyramidal side effects, and alcohol or other substance use).

Assess likelihood of dangerous or aggressive behavior, including potential for harm to others.

2. Psychiatric Management in the Acute Phase

Reduce overstimulating or stressful relationships, environments, and life events.

Provide the patient with information (appropriate to his or her ability to assimilate) on the nature and management of the illness.

Initiate a relationship with family members. Refer family members to local chapters of the National Alliance for the Mentally Ill (NAMI) and to the NAMI web site (www.nami.org).

3. Use of Antipsychotic Medications in the Acute Phase

Initiate antipsychotic medication as soon as it is feasible. It may be appropriate to delay pharmacologic treatment for patients who require more extensive diagnostic evaluation or who refuse medications or if psychosis is caused by substance use or acute stress reactions.

Discuss risks and benefits of the medication with the patient before initiating treatment, if feasible, and identify target symptoms (e.g., anxiety, poor sleep, hallucinations, and delusions) and acute side effects (e.g., orthostatic hypotension, dizziness, dystonic reactions, insomnia, and sedation).

Assess baseline levels of signs, symptoms, and laboratory values relevant to monitoring effects of antipsychotic therapy.
• Measure vital signs (pulse, blood pressure, temperature).
• Measure weight, height, and body mass index (BMI), which can be calculated with the formula weight in kilograms/(height in meters)^2 or the formula 703 × weight in pounds/(height in inches)^2 or with a BMI table:
     www.niddk.nih.gov/health/nutrit/pubs/statobes.htm#table
• Assess for extrapyramidal signs and abnormal involuntary movements.
• Screen for diabetes risk factors and measure fasting blood glucose.
• Screen for symptoms of hyperprolactinemia.
• Obtain lipid panel.
• Obtain ECG and serum potassium measurement before treatment with thioridazine, mesoridazine, or pimozide; obtain ECG before treatment with ziprasidone in the presence of cardiac risk factors.
• Conduct ocular examination, including slit-lamp examination, when beginning antipsychotics associated with increased risk of cataracts.
• Screen for changes in vision.
• Consider a pregnancy test for women with childbearing potential.

Minimize acute side effects (e.g., dystonia) that can influence willingness to accept and continue pharmacologic treatment.

Initiate rapid emergency treatments when an acutely psychotic patient is exhibiting aggressive behaviors toward self or others.
• Try talking to the patient in an attempt to calm him or her.
• Restraining the patient should be done only by a team trained in safe restraint procedures.
• Use short-acting parenteral formulations of first- or second-generation antipsychotic agents with or without parenteral benzodiazepine.
• Alternatively, use rapidly dissolving oral formulations of second-generation agents (e.g., olanzapine, risperidone) or oral concentrate formulations (e.g., risperidone, haloperidol).

See Tables 1 (p. 66) and 2 (p. 67) and Figure 1 (p. 68) for guidance in determining somatic treatment.

Select medication depending on the following factors:
• Prior degree of symptom response
• Past experience of side effects
• Side effect profile of prospective medications (see Table 3, p. 69)
• Patient's preferences for a particular medication, including route of administration
• Available formulations of medications (e.g., tablet, rapidly dissolving tablet, oral concentrate, short- and long-acting injection)

TABLE 1. Commonly Used Antipsychotic Medications

Antipsychotic Medication	Recommended Dose Range (mg/day)[a]	Chlorpromazine Equivalents (mg/day)[b]	Half-Life (hours)[c]
First-generation agents			
Phenothiazines			
Chlorpromazine	300–1000	100	6
Fluphenazine	5–20	2	33
Mesoridazine	150–400	50	36
Perphenazine	16–64	10	10
Thioridazine	300–800	100	24
Trifluoperazine	15–50	5	24
Butyrophenone			
Haloperidol	5–20	2	21
Others			
Loxapine	30–100	10	4
Molindone	30–100	10	24
Thiothixene	15–50	5	34
Second-generation agents			
Aripiprazole	10–30		75
Clozapine	150–600		12
Olanzapine	10–30		33
Quetiapine	300–800		6
Risperidone	2–8		24
Ziprasidone	120–200		7

[a]Dose range recommendations are adapted from the 2003 Schizophrenia Patient Outcome Research Team recommendations (Lehman AF, Kreyenbuhl J, Buchanan RW, et al.: "The Schizophrenia Patient Outcomes Research Team (PORT): Updated Treatment Recommendations 2003." *Schizophr Bull* [in press]).

[b]Chlorpromazine equivalents represent the approximate dose equivalent to 100 mg of chlorpromazine (relative potency). Chlorpromazine equivalents are not relevant to the second-generation antipsychotics; therefore, no chlorpromazine equivalents are indicated for these agents (Centorrino F, Eakin M, Bahk WM, et al.: "Inpatient Antipsychotic Drug Use in 1998, 1993, and 1989." *Am J Psychiatry* 159:1932–1935, 2002).

[c]The half-life of a drug is the amount of time required for the plasma drug concentration to decrease by one-half; half-life can be used to determine the appropriate dosing interval (Hardman JG, Limbird LE, Gilman AG (eds.): *Goodman and Gilman's The Pharmacological Basis of Therapeutics*, 10th ed. New York, McGraw-Hill Professional, 2001). The half-life of a drug does not include the half-life of its active metabolites.

TABLE 2. Choice of Medication in the Acute Phase of Schizophrenia

Patient Profile	Consider Medication From			
	Group 1: First-Generation Agents	Group 2: Risperidone, Olanzapine, Quetiapine, Ziprasidone, or Aripiprazole	Group 3: Clozapine	Group 4: Long-Acting Injectable Antipsychotic Agents
First episode		Yes		
Persistent suicidal ideation or behavior			Yes	
Persistent hostility and aggressive behavior			Yes	
Tardive dyskinesia		Yes; all group 2 drugs may not be equal in their lower or no tardive dyskinesia liability	Yes	
History of sensitivity to extrapyramidal side effects		Yes, except higher doses of risperidone		
History of sensitivity to prolactin elevation		Yes, except risperidone		
History of sensitivity to weight gain, hyperglycemia, or hyperlipidemia		Ziprasidone or aripiprazole		
Repeated nonadherence to pharmacological treatment				Yes

FIGURE 1. Somatic Treatment of Schizophrenia

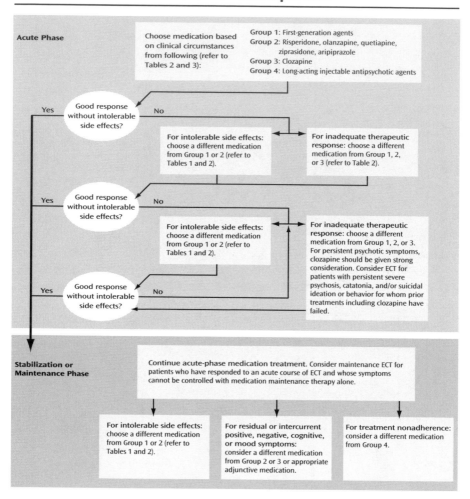

TABLE 3. Selected Side Effects of Commonly Used Antipsychotic Medications

Medication	Extra-pyramidal Side Effects/ Tardive Dyskinesia	Prolactin Elevation	Weight Gain	Glucose Abnormalities	Lipid Abnormalities	QTc Prolongation	Sedation	Hypotension	Anti-cholinergic Side Effects
Thioridazine	+	++	+	+?	+?	+++	++	++	++
Perphenazine	++	++	+	+?	+?	0	+	+	0
Haloperidol	+++	+++	+	0	0	0	++	0	0
Clozapine[a]	0[b]	0	+++	+++	+++	+	+++	+++	+++
Risperidone	+	+++	++	++	++	0	+	+	0
Olanzapine[b]	0[b]	0	+++	+++	+++	0	+	+	++
Quetiapine[c]	0[b]	0	++	++	++	0	++	++	0
Ziprasidone	0[b]	+	0	0	0	++	+	0	0
Aripiprazole[d]	0[b]	0	0	0	0	0	+	0	0

0 = No risk or rarely causes side effects at therapeutic dose. + = Mild or occasionally causes side effects at therapeutic dose. ++ = Sometimes causes side effects at therapeutic dose. +++ = Frequently causes side effects at therapeutic dose. ? = Data too limited to rate with confidence.

[a]Also causes agranulocytosis, seizures, and myocarditis.
[b]Possible exception of akathisia.
[c]Also carries warning about potential development of cataracts.
[d]Also causes nausea and headache.

Source. Adapted from Tandon R: "Antipsychotic Agents," in Current Psychotherapeutic Drugs, Second Edition. Edited by Quitkin FM, Adams DC, Bowden CL, et al. Philadelphia, PA, Current Medicine, 1998, pp. 120–154, with permission of Current Medicine, Inc.

3. Use of Antipsychotic Medications in the Acute Phase (continued)

Consider second-generation antipsychotics as first-line medications because of the decreased risk for extrapyramidal side effects and tardive dyskinesia.
- For patients who have had prior treatment success or who prefer first-generation agents, these medications are useful and for specific patients may be the first choice.
- With the possible exception of clozapine for patients with treatment-resistant symptoms, antipsychotics generally have similar efficacy in treating positive symptoms.
- Second-generation antipsychotics may have superior efficacy in treating global psychopathology and cognitive, negative, and mood symptoms.

Consider long-acting injectable antipsychotic medication for patients with recurrent relapses related to partial or full nonadherence. The oral form of the same medication (e.g., fluphenazine, haloperidol, and risperidone) is the logical choice for initial treatment.

Titrate as quickly as tolerated to the target therapeutic dose (sedation, orthostatic hypotension, and tachycardia are generally the side effects that limit the rate of increase), and monitor clinical status for at least 2 to 4 weeks.
- The optimal dose of first-generation antipsychotics is, for most patients, at the "extrapyramidal symptom (EPS) threshold," or the dose at which minimal rigidity is detectable on physical examination.
- For second-generation antipsychotics, target dose usually falls within the therapeutic dose range specified by the manufacturer and in the package labeling approved by the U.S. Food and Drug Administration.

If the patient is not improving, consider whether the lack of response can be explained by medication nonadherence, rapid medication metabolism, or poor medication absorption.

Consider measuring plasma concentration for those medications for which plasma concentration relates to clinical response (e.g., haloperidol, clozapine).

If the patient is adhering to treatment and has an adequate plasma concentration but is not responding to treatment, consider raising the dose for a finite period (if tolerated) or switching medications.

4. Use of Adjunctive Medications in the Acute Phase

Use adjunctive medications to treat comorbid conditions (e.g., major depression, obsessive-compulsive disorder) or associated symptoms (e.g., agitation, aggression, affective symptoms), to address sleep disturbances, and to treat antipsychotic drug side effects.

Be aware that some antidepressants (those that inhibit catecholamine reuptake) can potentially sustain or exacerbate psychotic symptoms in some individuals.

Benzodiazepines may be helpful for managing both anxiety and agitation during the acute phase of treatment.

Mood stabilizers and beta-blockers may be effective in reducing the severity of recurrent hostility and aggression.

4. Use of Adjunctive Medications in the Acute Phase (continued)

Consider the following factors when deciding on the prophylactic use of medications to treat extrapyramidal side effects:
- Propensity of the antipsychotic medication to cause extrapyramidal symptoms (Table 3, p. 69)
- Patient's preferences
- Patient's prior history of extrapyramidal symptoms
- Other risk factors for extrapyramidal symptoms (especially risk factors for dystonia)
- Risk factors for and potential consequences of anticholinergic side effects

Other potential strategies for treating extrapyramidal symptoms include lowering the dose of the antipsychotic medication or switching to a different antipsychotic medication.

5. Use of ECT and Other Somatic Therapies in the Acute Phase

Consider adding ECT to antipsychotic treatment for individuals with schizophrenia or schizoaffective disorder who have persistent severe psychosis and/or suicidal ideation or behaviors and for whom prior treatments, including clozapine, have failed.

Also consider ECT for individuals with prominent catatonic features that have not responded to an acute trial of lorazepam (e.g., 1 to 2 mg i.v. or i.m. or 2 to 4 mg p.o., repeated as needed over 48 to 72 hours).

For patients with schizophrenia and comorbid depression, ECT may also be beneficial if depressive symptoms are resistant to treatment or if features such as inanition or suicidal ideation or behavior, which necessitate a rapid response to treatment, are present.

6. Special Issues in Treatment of First-Episode Patients

Closely observe and document signs and symptoms over time, because a first episode of psychosis can be polymorphic and evolve into a variety of specific disorders (e.g., schizophreniform disorder, bipolar disorder, schizoaffective disorder).

More than 70% of first-episode patients achieve a full remission of psychotic signs and symptoms within 3 to 4 months, and more than 80% achieve stable remission at the end of 1 year. Predictors of poor treatment response include

- male gender,
- pre- or perinatal injury,
- more severe hallucinations and delusions,
- attentional impairments,
- poor premorbid function,
- longer duration of untreated psychosis,
- development of extrapyramidal side effects, and
- distressing emotional climate (e.g., hostile and critical attitudes and overprotection by others in one's living situation or high levels of expressed emotion).

Strive to minimize risk of relapse in a remitted patient, because of its clinical, social, and vocational costs (i.e., recurrent episodes are associated with increasing risk of chronic residual symptoms and evidence of neuroanatomical changes).

Aim to eliminate exposure to cannabinoids and psychostimulants, enhance stress management, and employ maintenance antipsychotic treatment.

6. Special Issues in Treatment of First-Episode Patients (continued)

Discuss candidly the high risk of relapse and factors that may minimize relapse risk. Prudent treatment options include 1) indefinite antipsychotic maintenance medication and 2) medication discontinuation with close follow-up and a plan of antipsychotic reinstitution with symptom recurrence.

C. Stabilization Phase

Goals of treatment
- Minimize stress on the patient and provide support to minimize the likelihood of relapse.
- Enhance the patient's adaptation to life in the community.
- Facilitate continued reduction in symptoms and consolidation of remission, and promote the process of recovery.

If the patient has achieved an adequate therapeutic response with minimal side effects, monitor response to the same medication and dose for the next 6 months.

Assess adverse side effects continuing from the acute phase, and adjust pharmacotherapy accordingly to minimize them.

Continue with supportive psychotherapeutic interventions.

Begin education for the patient (and continue education for family members) about the course and outcome of the illness and emphasize the importance of treatment adherence.

To avoid gaps in service delivery, arrange for linkage of services between hospital and community treatment before the patient is discharged from the hospital.

For hospitalized patients, it is frequently beneficial to arrange an appointment with an outpatient psychiatrist and, for patients who will reside in a community residence, to arrange a visit before discharge.

After discharge, help patients adjust to life in the community through realistic goal setting without undue pressure to perform at high levels vocationally and socially.

D. Stable Phase

Goals of treatment
- Ensure that symptom remission or control is sustained.
- Maintain or improve the patient's level of functioning and quality of life.
- Effectively treat increases in symptoms or relapses.
- Continue to monitor for adverse treatment effects.

1. Assessment in the Stable Phase

Ongoing monitoring and assessment are necessary to determine whether the patient might benefit from alterations in the treatment program.

Perform a clinical assessment for extrapyramidal symptoms (for patients taking antipsychotic medications) at each clinical visit.

1. Assessment in the Stable Phase *(continued)*

Perform a clinical assessment for abnormal involuntary movements every 6 months for patients taking first-generation antipsychotics and every 12 months for patients taking second-generation antipsychotics. For patients at increased risk (e.g., elderly patients), assessments should be made every 3 months and 6 months with treatment using first-generation and second-generation antipsychotics, respectively.

Monitor the patient's weight and BMI at each visit for 6 months and quarterly thereafter. For patients with BMI in the overweight (25 to 29.9 kg/m^2) or obese ($\geq$30 kg/m^2) range, routinely monitor for obesity-related health problems (e.g., blood pressure, serum lipids, clinical symptoms of diabetes).

Monitor fasting blood glucose or hemoglobin A1c at 4 months and then annually, and monitor other blood chemistries (e.g., electrolytes; renal, liver, and thyroid function) annually or as clinically indicated; consider drug toxicology screen if clinically indicated.

Depending on the specific medication being prescribed, consider other assessments, including vital signs, CBC, ECG, screening for symptoms of hyperprolactinemia, and ocular examination.

If the patient agrees, maintain strong ties with individuals who are likely to notice any resurgence of symptoms and the occurrence of life stresses and events.

2. Psychosocial Treatments in the Stable Phase

Select appropriate psychosocial treatments based on the circumstances of the individual patient's needs and social context.

Psychosocial treatments with demonstrated efficacy include
- family interventions,
- supported employment,
- assertive community treatment,
- social skills training, and
- cognitive behaviorally oriented psychotherapy.

3. Use of Antipsychotic Medications in the Stable Phase

Antipsychotics can reduce the risk of relapse in the stable phase of illness to less than 30% per year.

For most patients treated with first-generation antipsychotics, clinicians should prescribe a dose close to the "EPS threshold" (i.e., the dose that will induce extrapyramidal side effects with minimal rigidity detectable on physical examination).

Second-generation antipsychotics can generally be administered at doses that are therapeutic but that will not induce extrapyramidal side effects.

Weigh advantages of decreasing antipsychotics to the "minimal effective dose" against a somewhat greater risk of relapse and more frequent exacerbations of schizophrenia symptoms.

Evaluate whether residual negative symptoms are in fact secondary to a parkinsonian syndrome or an untreated major depressive syndrome, and treat accordingly.

4. Use of Adjunctive Medications in the Stable Phase

Add other psychoactive medication to antipsychotic medications in the stable phase to treat comorbid conditions, aggression, anxiety, or other mood symptoms; to augment the antipsychotic effects of the primary drug; and to treat side effects.

5. Use of ECT in the Stable Phase

Maintenance ECT may be helpful for some patients who have responded to acute treatment with ECT but for whom pharmacologic prophylaxis alone has been ineffective or cannot be tolerated.

6. Encourage the Patient and Family to Use Self-Help Treatment Organizations

E. Special Issues in Caring for Patients With Treatment-Resistant Illness

Carefully evaluate whether the patient has had an adequate trial of an antipsychotic, including whether the dose was adequate and whether the patient was taking the medication as prescribed.

Consider a trial of clozapine for a patient who has had what is considered a clinically inadequate response to two antipsychotics (at least one of which was a second-generation antipsychotic) and for a patient with persistent suicidal ideation or behavior that has not responded to other treatments.

Depending on the type of residual symptom (e.g., positive, negative, cognitive, or mood symptoms; aggressive behavior), augmentation strategies include adding another antipsychotic, anticonvulsants, or benzodiazepines.

ECT has demonstrated benefits in patients with treatment-resistant symptoms.

Cognitive behavior therapy techniques may have value in improving positive symptoms with low risk of side effects.

F. Treatment of Deficit Symptoms

Assess the patient for factors that may contribute to secondary negative symptoms.

If negative symptoms are secondary, treat their cause, e.g., antipsychotics for positive symptoms, antidepressants for depression, anxiolytics for anxiety disorders, or antiparkinsonian agents or antipsychotic dose reduction for extrapyramidal side effects.

If negative symptoms persist, they are presumed to be primary negative symptoms of the deficit state; although there are no treatments with proven efficacy, consider treatment with clozapine or other second-generation antipsychotics.

G. Choice of Treatment Setting or Housing

Indications for hospitalization usually include the patient's being considered to pose a serious threat of harm to self or others or being unable to care for self and needing constant supervision or support.

Other possible indications for hospitalization include general medical or psychiatric problems that make outpatient treatment unsafe or ineffective.

Legal proceedings to achieve involuntary hospitalization are indicated when patients decline voluntary status and hospitalization is clearly warranted.

Alternative treatment settings such as day or partial hospitalization, home care, family crisis therapy, crisis residential care, and assertive community treatment should be considered for patients who do not need formal hospitalization for their acute episodes but require more intensive services than can be expected in a typical outpatient setting.

Patients may be moved from one level of care to another on the basis of the factors described in Table 4 (p. 81).

TABLE 4. **Factors Affecting Choice of Treatment Setting or Housing**

Availability of the setting or housing

Patient's clinical condition
- Need for protection from harm to self or others
- Need for external structure and support
- Ability to cooperate with treatment

Patient's and family's preference

Requirements of the treatment plan
- Need for a particular treatment or a particular intensity of treatment that may be available only in certain settings
- Need for a specific treatment for a comorbid psychiatric or other general medical condition

Characteristics of the setting
- Degrees of support, structure, and restrictiveness
- Ability to protect patient from harm to self or others
- Availability of different treatment capacities, including general medical care and rehabilitation services
- Availability of psychosocial supports to facilitate the patient's receipt of treatment and to provide critical information to the psychiatrist about the patient's clinical status and response to treatments
- Capacity to care for severely agitated or psychotic patients
- Hours of operation
- Overall milieu and treatment philosophy

Patient's current environment or circumstances
- Family functioning
- Available social supports

TREATING MAJOR DEPRESSIVE DISORDER
A Quick Reference Guide

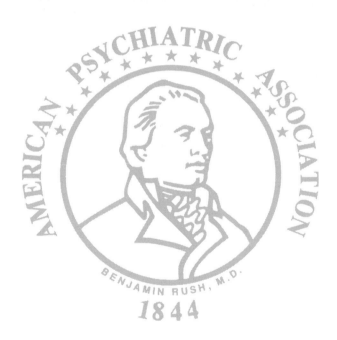

Based on *Practice Guideline for the Treatment of Patients With Major Depressive Disorder,*
Second Edition, originally published in April 2000. A guideline watch, summarizing significant
developments in the scientific literature since publication of this guideline, may be available
in the Psychiatric Practice section of the APA web site at www.psych.org.

OUTLINE

A. Psychiatric Management

Throughout the formulation of a treatment plan and all subsequent phases of treatment, the following principles of psychiatric management should be kept in mind:

1. Perform a diagnostic evaluation.

For general principles and components of a psychiatric evaluation, refer to APA's *Practice Guideline for the Psychiatric Evaluation of Adults.*

➤ Determine whether the diagnosis is depression.

➤ Determine whether there is psychiatric and general medical comorbidity.

➤ Include the following in the evaluation:
- History of the present illness and current symptoms
- Psychiatric history, including symptoms of mania
- Treatment history with current treatments and responses to previous treatments
- General medical history
- History of substance use disorders
- Personal history (e.g., psychological development, response to life transitions, major life events)
- Social, occupational, and family histories
- Review of the patient's medications
- Review of systems
- Mental status examination
- Physical examination
- Diagnostic tests as indicated

2. Evaluate the safety of the patient and others.

- Assessment of suicide risk is essential (see Table 1, p. 87).
- If the patient demonstrates suicidal or homicidal ideation, intention, or plans, close monitoring is required.
- Hospitalization should be considered if risk is significant.
- Note, however, that the ability to predict attempted or completed suicide is poor.

3. Evaluate and address functional impairments.

- Impairments include deficits in interpersonal relationships, work and living conditions, and other medical- or health-related needs.
- Address identified impairments (e.g., scheduling absences from work).

4. Determine the treatment setting.

Choose appropriate site, considering the following:
- Clinical condition (including symptom severity, comorbidity, suicidality, homicidality, and level of functioning)
- Available support systems
- Ability of the patient to adequately care for self, provide reliable feedback to the psychiatrist, and cooperate with treatment

Reevaluate optimal setting on an ongoing basis.

Consider hospitalization if the patient
- poses serious threat of harm to self or others (involuntary hospitalization may be necessary if patient refuses),
- is severely ill and lacks adequate social supports (alternatively, intensive day treatment may be appropriate),
- has certain comorbid psychiatric or general medical conditions, or
- has not responded adequately to outpatient treatment.

5. Establish and maintain a therapeutic alliance.

> - It is important to pay attention to the concerns of the patient and his or her family.
> - Be aware of transference and countertransference issues.

6. Monitor psychiatric status and safety.

> Monitor the patient for changes in destructive impulses to self and others.

> Be vigilant in monitoring changes in psychiatric status, including major depressive symptoms and symptoms of potential comorbid conditions.

> Consider diagnostic reevaluation if symptoms change significantly or if new symptoms emerge.

TABLE 1. **Considerations in the Evaluation for Suicide Risk**

- Presence of suicidal or homicidal ideation, intent, or plans
- Access to means for suicide and the lethality of those means
- Presence of psychotic symptoms, command hallucinations, or severe anxiety
- Presence of alcohol or substance use
- History and seriousness of previous attempts
- Family history of or recent exposure to suicide

7. Provide education to the patient and, when appropriate, to his or her family.

- Emphasize that major depressive disorder is a real illness.
- Education about treatments helps patients make informed decisions, be aware of side effects, and adhere to treatment.

8. Enhance medication adherence.

To improve adherence, emphasize
- when and how often to take medication,
- the typical 2- to 4-week lag for beneficial effects to be noticed,
- need to continue medication even after feeling better,
- need to consult with the prescribing doctor before medication discontinuation, and
- what to do if problems arise.

Improve adherence in elderly patients by simplifying the medication regimen and minimizing cost.

Consider psychotherapeutic intervention for serious or persistent nonadherence.

9. Address early signs of relapse.

Inform the patient (and, when appropriate, the family) about the significant risk of relapse.

Educate the patient (and the family) about how to identify early signs and symptoms of new episodes.

Emphasize seeking help if signs of relapse appear, to prevent full-blown exacerbation.

B. Acute Phase Treatment

1. Choice of Initial Treatment Modality (see Figure 1, p. 90)
a. Pharmacotherapy

Severity of Major Depressive Episode	Pharmacotherapy
Mild	Antidepressants if preferred by patient
Moderate to severe	Antidepressants are treatment of choice (unless electroconvulsive therapy [ECT] is planned)
With psychotic features	Antidepressants plus antipsychotics or ECT

Features suggesting that medication may be the preferred treatment include the following:
• History of prior positive response
• Severe symptomatology
• Significant sleep or appetite disturbances or agitation
• Anticipation of need for maintenance therapy
• Patient preference
• Lack of available alternative treatment modalities

FIGURE 1. Choice of Treatment Modalities for Major Depressive Disorder

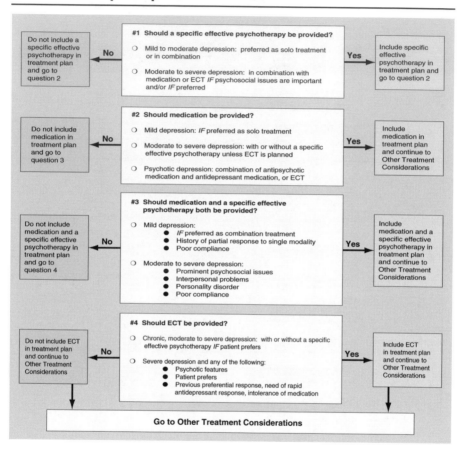

1. Choice of Initial Treatment Modality (see Figure 1, p. 90)
b. Psychotherapy Alone

If the severity of the major depressive episode is mild to moderate, use psychotherapy if preferred by the patient.

Features suggesting the use of psychotherapeutic interventions include the following:
• Presence of significant psychosocial stressors
• Intrapsychic conflict
• Interpersonal difficulties
• Comorbid personality disorder
• Pregnancy, lactation, or wish to become pregnant
• Patient preference

1. Choice of Initial Treatment Modality (see Figure 1, p. 90)
c. Combined Pharmacotherapy and Psychotherapy

Consider the use of combined pharmocotherapy and psychotherapy if the severity of the major depressive episode is mild to severe with clinically significant psychosocial issues, interpersonal problems, or a comorbid personality disorder.

Other features suggesting combination treatment include the following:
• History of only partial response to single treatment modalities
• Poor adherence to treatments (combine medication with a psychotherapeutic approach that focuses on treatment adherence)

1. Choice of Initial Treatment Modality (see Figure 1, p. 90)
d. Electroconvulsive Therapy

Consider ECT if any of the following features are present:
• Major depressive episode with a high degree of symptom severity and functional impairment
• Psychotic symptoms or catatonia
• Urgent need for response (e.g., suicidality or nutritional compromise in a patient refusing food)

ECT may be the preferred treatment when
• the presence of comorbid medical conditions precludes the use of antidepressant medications,
• there is a prior history of positive response to ECT, or
• the patient expresses a preference for ECT.

2. Choice of Antidepressant
a. Principles of Choosing an Initial Antidepressant

See Table 2 (p. 93) for a list of antidepressants and dosage ranges.

Because there is comparable efficacy between and within classes of medications, the initial selection is based largely on the following considerations:
• Anticipated side effects
• Safety or tolerability of side effects for individual patients
• Patient preference
• Quantity and quality of clinical trial data
• Cost

Based on these factors, the following medications are likely to be effective for most patients: selective serotonin reuptake inhibitors (SSRIs), desipramine, nortriptyline, bupropion, venlafaxine, nefazodone, and mirtazapine.

TABLE 2. Dosage Ranges for Antidepressant Medications

Generic Name	Starting Dosage (mg/day)[a]	Usual Dosage (mg/day)
Tricyclics and tetracyclics		
Tertiary amine tricyclics		
Amitriptyline	25–50	100–300
Clomipramine	25	100–250
Doxepin	25–50	100–300
Imipramine	25–50	100–300
Trimipramine	25–50	100–300
Secondary amine tricyclics		
Desipramine[b]	25–50	100–300
Nortriptyline[b]	25	50–150
Protriptyline	10	15–60
Tetracyclics		
Amoxapine	50	100–400
Maprotiline	50	100–225
SSRIs		
Citalopram[b]	20	20–60[c]
Fluoxetine[b]	20	20–60[c]
Fluvoxamine[b]	50	50–300[c]
Paroxetine[b]	20	20–50[c]
Sertraline[b]	50	50–200[c]
Dopamine-norepinephrine reuptake inhibitors		
Bupropion[b]	150	150–300
Bupropion, sustained release[b]	150	150–300
Serotonin-norepinephrine reuptake inhibitors		
Venlafaxine[b]	37.5	75–375
Venlafaxine, extended release[b]	37.5	75–225
Serotonin modulators		
Nefazodone	50	150–600
Trazodone	50	75–400
Norepinephrine-serotonin modulator		
Mirtazapine	15	15–45
MAOIs		
Irreversible, nonselective		
Phenelzine	15	15–90
Tranylcypromine	10	30–60

[a]Lower starting dosages are recommended for elderly patients and for patients with panic disorder, significant anxiety or hepatic disease, and general comorbidity.
[b]These medications are likely to be optimal medications in terms of the patient's acceptance of side effects, safety, and quantity and quality of clinical trial data.
[c]Dose varies with diagnosis; see text for specific guidelines.

2. Choice of Antidepressant
a. Principles of Choosing an Initial Antidepressant (continued)

Consider other features, including the following:
- History of prior response with a particular antidepressant
- Presence of comorbid psychiatric or general medical conditions (e.g., tertiary amine tricyclic antidepressants [TCAs] may not be optimal in patients with cardiovascular conditions or acute-angle glaucoma)

Use monoamine oxidase inhibitors (MAOIs) only for patients who do not respond to other treatments, because of MAOIs' dietary restrictions and potentially serious side effects.
- MAOIs may be particularly effective for major depressive episodes with atypical features (although in clinical practice, SSRIs are now commonly used for atypical depression because of their more favorable adverse effect profile).

2. Choice of Antidepressant
b. Implementation of Antidepressant Therapy

Start at the dosage levels suggested in Table 2 (p. 93).

Titrate to full therapeutic dosage, taking the following considerations into account:
- Side effects
- Patient's age
- Comorbid illnesses (e.g., starting and therapeutic doses should be reduced [generally to half] in elderly or medically frail patients)

Monitor to assess the following:
- Treatment response
- Side effects (see Figure 2, below)
- Clinical condition
- Safety (e.g., suicidality)

Determine the monitoring frequency. Frequency depends on
- severity of illness,
- suicide risk,
- significant side effects or drug interactions,
- patient's cooperation with treatment,
- availability of social supports, and
- presence of comorbid general medical problems.

Determine the method of monitoring (face-to-face, phone, or e-mail contact, contact with a physician knowledgeable about the patient) according to clinical context.

FIGURE 2. **Management of Medication Side Effects**

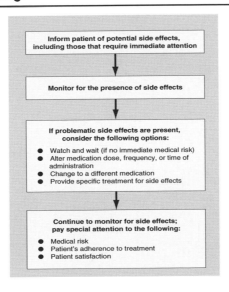

2. Choice of Antidepressant
c. Initial Failure to Respond

➤ If the patient is not at least moderately improved after 4 to 8 weeks, reappraise the treatment regimen (see Figure 3, p. 97).

➤ Investigate the patient's adherence to treatment.

➤ Consider pharmacokinetic/pharmacodynamic factors (may require serum antidepressant medication levels).

➤ Revise the treatment plan and consider the following options:
- Maximize the initial therapeutic treatment dose.
  - For partial responders, extend the trial (e.g., by 2 to 4 weeks).
  - For nonresponders on moderate doses or those with low serum levels, raise the dose and monitor for increased side effects.
- Add, change, or increase the frequency of psychotherapy.
- Switch to another non-MAOI medication (see Table 2, p. 93, and Table 3, p. 98) in either the same class or a different class, particularly if there is lack of partial response.
- Especially if there is partial response, augment with
  - a non-MAOI antidepressant from a different class (be alert to drug-drug interactions), or
  - another adjuvant medication (e.g., lithium, thyroid hormone, anticonvulsants, psychostimulants).
- Switch to an MAOI.
- Institute ECT.

FIGURE 3. Acute Phase Treatment of Major Depressive Disorder

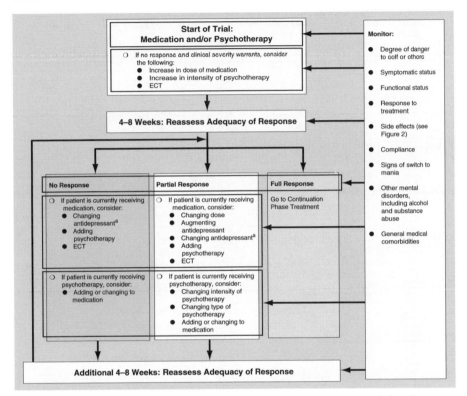

[a]Choose either another antidepressant from the same class or, if two previous medication trials from the same class were ineffective, an antidepressant from a different class.

TABLE 3. **Required Washout Times Between Antidepressant Trials**

Antidepressant Change	Minimum Washout Period
To MAOI from drug with long–half-life metabolites (e.g., fluoxetine)	5 weeks
To MAOI from drug without long–half-life metabolites (e.g., TCA, paroxetine, fluvoxamine, venlafaxine) or other MAOI	2 weeks
To non-MAOI antidepressant from MAOI	2 weeks

2. Choice of Antidepressant
d. Continued Failure to Respond

Verify the patient's diagnosis and adherence to treatment.

If the patient does not show at least moderate improvement after an additional 4 to 8 weeks, explore the presence of other factors that might interfere with improvement:
• Comorbid general medical conditions
• Comorbid psychiatric disorders (including substance abuse)
• Significant psychosocial problems

If the steps above do not clarify the reason for the nonresponse, consider consultation or possibly ECT.

3. Choice of Psychotherapy
a. Principles of Choosing a Psychotherapy

Choose the modality of therapy:
- Cognitive behavior therapy and interpersonal therapy have the best research-documented efficacy.
- Psychodynamic psychotherapy, supported by broad clinical consensus, is usually oriented toward both symptomatic improvement and broader personality issues.

Consider other factors:
- Patient preference
- Availability of clinicians with appropriate training and expertise in the specific approach

3. Choice of Psychotherapy
b. Psychotherapy Implementation

Determine the frequency of psychotherapy.
Frequency generally ranges from once to several times per week in the acute phase and depends on
- specific type and goals of psychotherapy,
- need to create and maintain a therapeutic relationship,
- need to ensure treatment adherence, and
- need to monitor and address suicidality.

In situations with more than one treating clinician, maintain ongoing contact with the patient and other clinicians.

If the patient does not show at least moderate improvement after 4 to 8 weeks, conduct a thorough review and reappraisal (see Figure 3, p. 97).

4. Choice of Medication Plus Psychotherapy

Consider the same issues that influence the choice of medication (see section B.2, p. 92) and psychotherapy (see section B.3, p. 99).

If the patient does not show at least moderate improvement after 4 to 8 weeks, conduct a thorough review, including of adherence and pharmacokinetic/pharmacodynamic factors.

If the patient does not show at least moderate improvement after an additional 4 to 8 weeks following a change, conduct another thorough review and consider consultation or possibly ECT.

5. Assessing Adequacy of Treatment Response

Do not conclude acute phase treatment if the patient shows only partial response. Partial response is associated with poor functional outcome.

C. Continuation Phase

The continuation phase is defined as the 16- to 20-week period after sustained and complete remission from the acute phase.

To prevent relapse, continue antidepressant medication at the same dose used during the acute phase.

Consider the use of psychotherapy to help prevent relapse.

Consider providing ECT if medication or psychotherapy has not been effective.

Set frequency of visits depending on clinical condition and specific treatments used. Frequency can vary from once every 2 to 3 months to multiple times per week.

D. Maintenance Phase

The goal during the maintenance phase is to prevent recurrences of major depressive episodes (see Table 4, p. 102, for factors to consider).

Continue using the treatment that was effective in the acute and continuation phases.

Employ the same full antidepressant medication dosages used in prior phases of treatment.

Set the frequency of visits according to clinical condition and specific treatments used.
Frequency can range from as low as once every 2 to 3 months for stable patients to as high as multiple times per week for those in psychodynamic psychotherapy.

Consider ECT maintenance for patients who have repeated moderate or severe episodes despite adequate pharmacological treatment (or who are unable to tolerate maintenance medication).

TABLE 4. Considerations in the Decision to
Use Maintenance Treatment

Factor	Component
Risk of recurrence	Number of prior episodes; presence of comorbid conditions; residual symptoms between episodes
Severity of episodes	Suicidality; psychotic features; severe functional impairments
Side effects experienced with continuous treatment	
Patient preferences	

E. Discontinuation of Active Treatment

Consider whether to discontinue treatment based on the same factors considered in the decision to initiate maintenance treatment.
For example, consider the probability of recurrence and the frequency and severity of past episodes (see Table 4, above, and Table 5, p. 103).

When discontinuing psychotherapy, the best method depends on the patient's needs and type of psychotherapy, the duration of treatment, and the intensity of treatment.

To discontinue pharmacotherapy, taper the dose over at least several weeks.
• Facilitates more rapid return to a full dose if symptoms recur.
• Minimizes the risk of antidepressant discontinuation syndromes (more likely with shorter–half-life antidepressants).

> Establish a plan to restart treatment in case of relapse.

> If the patient experiences a relapse when medication is discontinued, resume the previously successful treatment.

TABLE 5. Risk Factors for Recurrence of Major Depressive Disorder

- Prior history of multiple episodes of major depressive disorder
- Persistence of dysthymic symptoms after recovery from an episode of major depressive disorder
- Presence of an additional, nonaffective psychiatric diagnosis
- Presence of a chronic general medical condition

TREATING
BIPOLAR DISORDER
A Quick Reference Guide

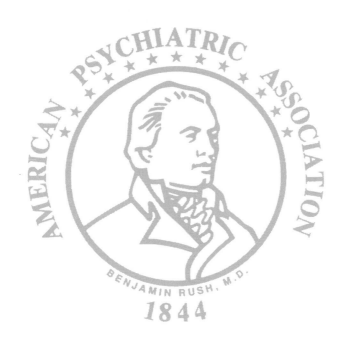

Based on *Practice Guideline for the Treatment of Patients With Bipolar Disorder,* Second Edition, originally published in April 2002. A guideline watch, summarizing significant developments in the scientific literature since publication of this guideline, may be available in the Psychiatric Practice section of the APA web site at www.psych.org.

OUTLINE

A. Psychiatric Management

Goals of Psychiatric Management
- Establish and maintain a therapeutic alliance.
- Monitor the patient's psychiatric status.
- Provide education regarding bipolar disorder.
- Enhance treatment adherence.
- Promote regular patterns of activity and sleep.
- Anticipate stressors.
- Identify new episodes early.
- Minimize functional impairments.

1. Perform a diagnostic evaluation.

Assess for the presence of an alcohol or substance use disorder or other factors that may contribute to the disease process or complicate its treatment.
- Neurological conditions commonly associated with secondary mania are multiple sclerosis and lesions involving right-sided subcortical structures or cortical areas closely linked to the limbic system.
- L-Dopa and corticosteroids are the most common medications associated with secondary mania.
- Substance use may precipitate mood episodes. Patients may also use substances to ameliorate the symptoms of such episodes.

Inquire about a history of time periods with mood dysregulation or lability accompanied by associated manic symptoms (e.g., decreased sleep).
- Bipolar disorder commonly presents with depressive symptoms.
- Patients rarely volunteer information about manic or hypomanic symptoms.

2. Ensure the safety of the patient and others and determine a treatment setting.

Evaluate safety.
- Careful assessment of the patient's risk for suicide is critical; lifetime rates of completed suicide for people with bipolar disorder are as high as 10% to 15%.
- The overwhelming majority of suicide attempts are associated with depressive episodes or depressive features during mixed episodes.
- Ask every patient about suicidal ideation, intention to act on these ideas, and extent of plans or preparation for suicide.
- Collect collateral information from family members or others.
- Assess for access to means of committing suicide (e.g., medications, firearms) and the lethality of these means.
- Assess for factors associated with increased risk, such as agitation, pervasive insomnia, impulsiveness, or other psychiatric comorbidity such as substance abuse, psychosis (especially with command hallucinations), or personality disorder.
- Assess for family history of suicide and history of recent exposure to suicide.
- Consider the nature and potential lethality of any prior suicide attempts.
- Closely monitor patients who exhibit suicidal or violent ideas or intent.
- Carefully document your decision-making process.

Consider hospitalization for patients who
- pose a serious threat of harm to themselves or others,
- are severely ill and lack adequate social support outside a hospital setting or demonstrate significantly impaired judgment,
- have complicating psychiatric or general medical conditions, or
- have not responded adequately to outpatient treatment.

Reevaluate the treatment setting on an ongoing basis to determine whether it is optimal or whether the patient would benefit more from a different level of care.

Provide a calm and highly structured environment.

Consider limiting access to cars, credit cards, bank accounts, or telephones and cellular phones during the manic phase because of the risk of reckless behavior.

3. Establish and maintain a therapeutic alliance.

- A therapeutic alliance is critical for understanding and managing the individual patient.
- Over time, knowledge gained about the patient and the illness course allows early identification of usual prodromal symptoms and early recognition of new episodes.

4. Monitor the patient's psychiatric status.

- Monitoring is especially important during manic episodes, when patient insight is often limited or absent.
- Be aware that small changes in mood or behavior may herald the onset of an episode.

5. Educate the patient and his or her family.

- Be aware that, over time, patients will vary in their ability to understand and retain information and accept and adapt to the need for long-term treatment.
- Education should be an ongoing process in which the psychiatrist gradually but persistently introduces facts about the illness and its treatment.
- Printed and Internet material (e.g., from www.psych.org) can be helpful.
- Use similar educational approaches for family members and significant others.

6. Enhance treatment adherence.

- Ambivalence about treatment is often expressed as poor adherence to medication or other treatments.
- Causes of ambivalence include
  - lack of insight about having a serious illness and
  - reluctance to give up the experience of hypomania or mania.
- Medication side effects, cost, and other demands of long-term treatment may be burdensome and need to be discussed.
- Many side effects can be corrected with careful attention to dosing, scheduling, and medication formulation (e.g., sustained release, liquid).

7. Promote awareness of stressors and regular patterns of activity and sleep.

- Stressors commonly precede episodes in all phases of the illness.
- Social rhythm disruption with disrupted sleep-wake cycles may specifically trigger manic episodes.
- Patients and their families should be informed about the potential effects of sleep disruption in triggering manic episodes.
- Regular patterns for daily activities should be promoted, including sleeping, eating, physical activity, and social and emotional stimulation.

8. Work with the patient to anticipate and address early signs of relapse.

- The psychiatrist should help the patient, family members, and significant others recognize early signs and symptoms of manic or depressive episodes.
- Early markers of episode onset are often predictable across episodes for an individual patient.
- Early identification of a prodrome is facilitated by the psychiatrist's consistent relationship with the patient as well as with the patient's family.

9. Evaluate and manage functional impairments.

Identify and address impairments in functioning.
- Assist the patient in scheduling absences from work or other responsibilities.
- Encourage the patient to avoid major life changes while in a depressive or manic state.
- Assess and address the needs of children of patients with bipolar disorder.

B. Treatment Options

1. Acute Manic or Mixed Episodes

Goals of Treatment
- Control symptoms to allow a return to usual levels of psychosocial functioning.
- Rapidly control agitation, aggression, and impulsivity.

Choose an initial treatment modality.

For patients not yet in treatment for bipolar disorder:

For *severe mania or mixed episodes,* initiate lithium in combination with an antipsychotic or valproate in combination with an antipsychotic.

For *less ill patients,* monotherapy with lithium, valproate, or an antipsychotic such as olanzapine may be sufficient.

- Short-term adjunctive treatment with a benzodiazepine may also be helpful.
- For mixed episodes, valproate may be preferred over lithium.
- Atypical antipsychotics are preferred over typical antipsychotics because of their generally more tolerable side effect profile (most current evidence supports the use of olanzapine and risperidone).
- Alternatives include 1) carbamazepine or oxcarbazepine in lieu of lithium or valproate and 2) ziprasidone or quetiapine in lieu of another antipsychotic.
- Treatment selection depends on illness severity, associated features such as rapid cycling or psychosis, and, where possible, patient preference.
- Antidepressants should be tapered and discontinued if possible.
- Psychosocial therapies and pharmacotherapies should be combined.

For patients who suffer a "breakthrough" manic or mixed episode while on maintenance treatment, optimize the medication dose.

- Ensure that serum levels are within the therapeutic range; in some instances, achieve a higher serum level (but still within the therapeutic range).
- Introduction or resumption of an antipsychotic is often necessary.
- Severely ill or agitated patients may also require short-term adjunctive treatment with a benzodiazepine.

If symptoms are inadequately controlled within 10 to 14 days of treatment with optimized doses of the first-line medication regimen, add another first-line medication.

- Alternative treatment options include adding carbamazepine or oxcarbazepine in lieu of an additional first-line medication (lithium, valproate, antipsychotic), adding an antipsychotic if not already prescribed, or changing from one antipsychotic to another.
- Clozapine may be particularly effective in refractory illness.
- Electroconvulsive therapy (ECT) may also be considered for
  - manic patients who are severely ill or whose mania is treatment resistant;
  - patients who, after consultation with the psychiatrist, prefer ECT;
  - patients with mixed episodes; and
  - patients with severe mania during pregnancy.

For psychosis during a manic or mixed episode, treat with an antipsychotic medication.

- Atypical antipsychotics are favored because of their generally more tolerable side effect profile.
- ECT may also be considered.

2. Acute Depression

Goals of Treatment
• Achieve remission of the symptoms of major depression and return the patient to usual levels of psychosocial functioning.
• Avoid precipitating a manic or hypomanic episode.

Choose an initial treatment modality.

For patients not yet in treatment for bipolar disorder, initiate either lithium or lamotrigine.
• As an alternative, especially for more severely ill patients, consider initiating treatment with both lithium and an antidepressant simultaneously (although supporting data are limited).
• Antidepressant monotherapy is not recommended.
• Consider ECT for
  - patients with life-threatening inanition, suicidality, or psychosis or
  - severe depression during pregnancy.
• Treatment selection should be guided by illness severity, associated features such as rapid cycling or psychosis, and, where possible, patient preference.
• Interpersonal therapy and cognitive behavior therapy may be useful when added to pharmacotherapy.
• Although psychodynamic psychotherapy for bipolar depression has not been empirically studied, it is widely used in combination with medication.

For patients who suffer a breakthrough depressive episode while on maintenance treatment, optimize the medication dosage.
Ensure that serum levels are within the therapeutic range; in some instances, achieve a higher serum level (but still within the therapeutic range).

If the patient fails to respond to optimized maintenance treatment, consider adding lamotrigine, bupropion, or paroxetine.
- Alternative next steps include adding another newer antidepressant (e.g., another selective serotonin reuptake inhibitor [SSRI] or venlafaxine) or a monoamine oxidase inhibitor (MAOI).
- Tricyclic antidepressants may carry a greater risk of precipitating a switch and are not recommended.
- MAOIs may be difficult to use because of the risk of severe drug and dietary interactions.
- Psychotic features during depression usually require adjunctive treatment with an antipsychotic medication.
- Consider ECT for
  - severe or treatment-resistant depression,
  - psychotic features, or
  - catatonic features.
- Clinicians may elect to use antidepressants earlier for bipolar II depression than for bipolar I depression because patients with bipolar II disorder probably have lower rates of antidepressant-induced switching into hypomania or mania.

3. Rapid Cycling

Identify and treat medical conditions such as hypothyroidism or drug or alcohol use that may contribute to cycling.

If possible, taper medications (particularly antidepressants) that may contribute to cycling.

For initial treatment, include lithium or valproate.
- An alternative treatment is lamotrigine.
- For many patients, combinations of medications are required (i.e., combining two of the agents above or one of them plus an antipsychotic).

4. Maintenance

Goals of Treatment
• Prevent relapse and recurrence.
• Reduce subthreshold symptoms.
• Reduce suicide risk.
• Reduce cycling frequency or milder degrees of mood instability.
• Improve overall function.

Determine whether maintenance treatment is indicated.
• Maintenance medication is recommended following a manic or a depressive episode.
• Although few maintenance studies of bipolar II disorder have been conducted, maintenance treatment warrants strong consideration for this form of the illness.

Choose an initial treatment modality.

Recommended options
• Treatment options with the best empirical support include lithium or valproate. Possible alternatives include lamotrigine, carbamazepine, or oxcarbazepine.
• If one of the above medications led to remission from the most recent depressive or manic episode, it generally should be continued.
• Maintenance ECT may also be considered for patients who respond to ECT during an acute episode.
• Treatment selection should be guided by illness severity, associated features such as rapid cycling or psychosis, and, where possible, patient preference.

Role of antipsychotics
- Antipsychotic medications should be discontinued unless they are needed for control of persistent psychosis or prevention of recurrence of mood episodes.
- Although maintenance therapy with atypical antipsychotics may be considered, there is as yet no definitive evidence that their efficacy in maintenance treatment is comparable to that of the other agents discussed above.

Role of psychosocial interventions
- Concomitant psychosocial interventions addressing illness management (i.e., adherence, lifestyle changes, and early detection of prodromal symptoms) and interpersonal difficulties are likely to be of benefit.
- Supportive and psychodynamic psychotherapies are widely used in combination with medication.
- Group psychotherapy and family therapy may also help patients address issues such as adherence to a treatment plan, adaptation to a chronic illness, regulation of self-esteem, and management of marital and other psychosocial issues.
- Support groups provide useful information about bipolar disorder and its treatment.

If the patient fails to respond (i.e., continues to experience subthreshold symptoms or breakthrough mood episodes), add another maintenance medication, an atypical antipsychotic, or an antidepressant.
- There are insufficient data to support one combination over another.
- Maintenance ECT may also be considered for patients who respond to ECT during an acute episode.

C. Additional Information About Pharmacotherapeutic Agents

1. Lithium

Side effects
- Up to 75% of patients experience some side effects, but most side effects either are minor or can be reduced or eliminated by lowering the lithium dose or changing the dosage schedule.
- Side effects related to peak serum levels (e.g., tremor within 1 to 2 hours of a dose) may be reduced or eliminated by using a slow-release preparation or changing to a single bedtime dose.
- Side effects include polyuria, polydypsia, weight gain, cognitive problems, tremor, sedation or lethargy, impaired coordination, gastrointestinal distress, hair loss, benign leukocytosis, acne, and edema.
- With long-term lithium treatment (>10 years), 10% to 20% of patients display morphological kidney changes. These changes are not generally associated with renal failure, although there are some case reports of renal insufficiency probably induced by lithium.
- Most patients experience some toxic effects with levels above 1.5 meq/L; levels above 2.0 meq/L are commonly associated with life-threatening side effects. At higher serum levels, hemodialysis may be needed to minimize toxicity.

Implementation

Initial workup
The following are generally recommended before beginning lithium therapy:
- General medical history and physical examination
- Blood urea nitrogen (BUN) and creatinine levels
- Tests of thyroid function
- Electrocardiogram (ECG) with rhythm strip for patients over age 40
- Pregnancy test (in women of childbearing age)

Dosing
- Start in low divided dosages to minimize side effects (e.g., 300 mg t.i.d. or less, depending on the patient's weight and age).
- Titrate dosage upward (generally to serum concentrations of 0.5 to 1.2 meq/L) according to response and side effects.
- Check lithium level after each dosage increase (steady-state levels are likely to be reached approximately 5 days after a dosage adjustment).
- Check at shorter intervals after dosage increase as levels approach upper limits of the therapeutic range (i.e., greater than 1.0 meq/L).
- The "optimal" maintenance level may vary from patient to patient. Some patients require the level used to treat acute mania; others can be satisfactorily maintained at lower levels.

Long-term monitoring of laboratory values
- Serum lithium levels
  - At minimum, check every 6 months in stable patients and whenever the clinical status changes.
  - The optimal frequency of monitoring depends on the stability of lithium levels over time for that patient and the degree to which the patient can be relied on to notice and report symptoms.
- Renal function
  - In general, during the first 6 months of treatment, test every 2 to 3 months.
  - Subsequently, check every 6 to 12 months in stable patients as well as whenever the clinical status changes.
- Thyroid function
  - In general, during the first 6 months of treatment, test once or twice.
  - Subsequently, check every 6 to 12 months in stable patients and whenever the clinical status changes.

2. Divalproex/Valproate/Valproic Acid

Side effects
- Common dose-related side effects of valproate include gastrointestinal distress, benign hepatic transaminase elevations, osteoporosis, tremor, and sedation.
- Patients with past or current hepatic disease may be at increased risk for hepatotoxicity.
- Mild, asymptomatic leukopenia and thrombocytopenia occur less frequently and are reversible on drug discontinuation.
- Other side effects include hair loss, increased appetite, and weight gain.
- Although risks are unclear, female patients should be monitored for possible development of polycystic ovarian syndrome.
- Rare, idiosyncratic, but potentially fatal adverse events include irreversible hepatic failure, hemorrhagic pancreatitis, and agranulocytosis; patients should be educated about the signs and symptoms of hepatic and hematological dysfunction and warned to contact their physician immediately if symptoms develop.

Implementation

Initial workup
The following are generally recommended before beginning valproate therapy:
- Before treatment, take a general medical history with special attention to hepatic, hematological, and bleeding abnormalities.
- Obtain liver function tests and hematological measures.

Dosing
- For hospitalized patients with acute mania, valproate can be administered at an initial dosage of 20 to 30 mg/kg per day in inpatients. After obtaining a valproate level, adjust the dose to achieve a serum level between 50 and 125 µg/mL.
- For outpatients, elderly patients, or patients with hypomania or euthymia, start at 250 mg t.i.d. Titrate the dose upward by 250 to 500 mg/day every few days, depending on clinical response and side effects, generally to a serum concentration of 50 to 125 µg/mL, with a maximum adult daily dosage of 60 mg/kg per day. Once the patient is stable, simplify to once- or twice-daily dosing.
- Bioavailability of the extended-release preparation, divalproex ER, is about 15% less than that of the immediate-release preparation; doses of divalproex ER will need to be increased proportionately.

Drug interactions
- Valproate displaces highly protein-bound drugs from their protein binding sites. Dosage adjustments will be needed.
- Because valproate inhibits lamotrigine metabolism, lamotrigine must be initiated at less than half the usual dose.

Long-term monitoring of laboratory values
- Patients should be educated about the signs and symptoms of hepatic and hematological dysfunction and instructed to report these symptoms if they occur.
- Most psychiatrists perform clinical assessments, including tests of hematological and hepatic function, at a minimum of every 6 months for stable patients who are taking valproate.
- Serum levels of valproic acid should be checked when clinically indicated (e.g., when another medication may change the metabolism of valproic acid).

3. Carbamazepine

Side effects

- Up to 50% of patients receiving carbamazepine experience side effects.
- The most common side effects include fatigue, nausea, and neurological symptoms such as diplopia, blurred vision, and ataxia.
- Less frequent side effects include skin rashes, mild leukopenia, mild liver enzyme elevations, mild thrombocytopenia, hyponatremia, and (less commonly) hypo-osmolality.
- Rare, idiosyncratic, but serious and potentially fatal side effects include agranulocytosis, aplastic anemia, thrombocytopenia, hepatic failure, exfoliative dermatitis (e.g., Stevens-Johnson syndrome), and pancreatitis.
- In addition to careful monitoring of clinical status, it is essential to educate patients about the signs and symptoms of hepatic, hematological, or dermatological reactions and instruct them to report symptoms if they occur.
- Other rare side effects include systemic hypersensitivity reactions; cardiac conduction disturbances; psychiatric symptoms, including sporadic cases of psychosis; and, very rarely, renal effects, including renal failure, oliguria, hematuria, and proteinuria.
- The carbamazepine analogue oxcarbazepine may be a useful alternative to carbamazepine based on its superior side effect profile.

Implementation

Initial workup
The following are generally recommended before beginning carbamazepine therapy:
- Minimum baseline evaluation should include a complete blood count (CBC) with differential and platelet count, a liver profile (LDH, SGOT, SGPT, bilirubin, alkaline phosphatase), and renal function tests. Serum electrolytes may also be obtained, especially in the elderly, who may be at higher risk for hyponatremia.
- Before treatment, a general medical history and a physical examination should be done, with special emphasis on prior history of blood dyscrasias or liver disease.

Dosing
- Carbamazepine is usually begun at a total daily dose of 200 to 600 mg, in three to four divided doses.
- In hospitalized patients with acute mania, the dosage may be increased in increments of 200 mg/day up to 800 to 1000 mg/day (unless side effects develop), with slower increases thereafter as indicated.
- In less acutely ill outpatients, dose adjustments should be slower to minimize side effects.
- Maintenance dosages average about 1000 mg/day but may range from 200 to 1600 mg/day in routine clinical practice.
- Levels established for treatment of seizure disorders (serum concentration between 4 and 12 µg/mL) are generally applied to patients with bipolar disorder.
- Use trough levels (drawn prior to the first morning dose) 5 days after a dose change.

3. Carbamazepine

Implementation *(continued)*

Long-term monitoring of laboratory values
- CBC, platelet, and liver function tests should be performed every 2 weeks during the first 2 months of carbamazepine treatment.
- Thereafter, if laboratory tests remain normal and no symptoms of bone marrow suppression or hepatitis appear, blood counts and liver function tests should be obtained at least every 3 months; more frequent monitoring is necessary if there are hematological or hepatic abnormalities.

4. Olanzapine

Side effects
- Common side effects include somnolence, constipation, dry mouth, increased appetite, and weight gain.
- During initial dose titration, olanzapine may induce orthostatic hypotension associated with dizziness, tachycardia, and in some patients, syncope.

Implementation
- For inpatients with acute mania, a starting dosage of 15 mg/day is suggested.
- For outpatients, lower starting dosages of 5 to 10 mg/day may be indicated.

5. Lamotrigine

Side effects
- The most common side effects are headache, nausea, infection, and xerostomia.
- In early clinical trials with patients with epilepsy, rapid titration of lamotrigine dosage was associated with a risk of serious rash, including Stevens-Johnson syndrome and toxic epidermal necrolysis. Risk was approximately 0.3% in adults and approximately 1% in children.
- Patients should be informed of the risk of rash and of the need to contact the psychiatrist or primary care physician immediately if any rash occurs.
- Rash can occur at any time during treatment but is more likely early in treatment.
- At rash onset, it is difficult to distinguish between a serious and a more benign rash.
- Particularly worrisome, however, are rashes accompanied by fever or sore throat, those that are diffuse and widespread, and those with prominent facial or mucosal involvement. In such circumstances, lamotrigine (and valproate, if administered concurrently) should be discontinued.
- In clinical trials, use of a slow dosage titration schedule (see below) reduced the risk of serious rash in adults to 0.01% (comparable to other anticonvulsants).
- Rash may be more likely if lamotrigine and valproate are administered concomitantly.

Implementation
- Lamotrigine should be administered at 25 mg/day for the first 2 weeks, then at 50 mg for weeks 3 and 4.
- After that, 50 mg/week can be added as clinically indicated.
- To minimize the risk of potentially serious rash in patients who are receiving valproate, the dose or the dosage schedule should be halved (i.e., 12.5 mg/day or 25 mg every other day for 2 weeks, then 25 mg daily for weeks 3 and 4).
- Concurrent carbamazepine treatment will lead to increased metabolism of lamotrigine and will require that dosing be doubled.

TREATING PANIC DISORDER
A Quick Reference Guide

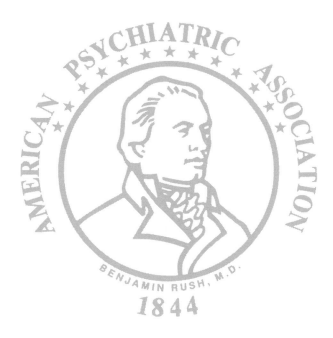

Based on *Practice Guideline for the Treatment of Patients With Panic Disorder,*
originally published in May 1998. A guideline watch, summarizing significant developments
in the scientific literature since publication of this guideline, may be available in the
Psychiatric Practice section of the APA web site at www.psych.org.

OUTLINE

A. Formulation and Implementation of a Treatment Plan

1. Treatment Setting

Outpatient treatment is indicated for most patients.

Consider hospitalization for the following indications:
• Comorbid depression, especially in patients who are at risk of suicide attempts
• Comorbid substance use disorders, especially in patients who require detoxification

2. Evaluation

Perform a comprehensive general medical and psychiatric evaluation.
• Follow principles of APA's *Practice Guideline for the Psychiatric Evaluation of Adults.*
• Determine whether diagnosis of panic disorder is warranted.
• Assess for comorbid psychiatric or general medical conditions.
• Consider general medical conditions and substance or medication use as causes of panic symptoms, especially in patients with new onset of symptoms.
• Perform indicated diagnostic studies and laboratory tests.

3. Treatment Modalities

Consider efficacy, risks and benefits, costs, and patient preference in choice of modality.
- Panic-focused cognitive behavior therapy (CBT) and medications have both been shown to be effective treatments for panic disorder.
- There is no evidence for superiority of either CBT or medications. Rather, choice of modality is mainly determined by weighing advantages and disadvantages (see Appendix A in this guide, p. 140).
- Psychodynamic or other psychotherapies may be the treatment of choice for some patients.
- Combined psychosocial and pharmacological treatments may have advantages over either modality alone.

Choose treatment modalities to be used in conjunction with psychiatric management.
See section C (p. 137) for more detail about specific modalities.

Psychotherapies
- Panic-focused CBT is generally administered in weekly sessions for approximately 12 weeks.
- CBT approaches can be conducted in group formats.
- Psychodynamic psychotherapy may be useful in reducing symptoms or maladaptive behaviors in patients with complicating comorbid axis I and axis II conditions.
- Consider employing family and supportive therapy along with other psychosocial and pharmacological treatments.
- Sessions that include significant others help to relieve stress on families and may facilitate adherence.
- Psychotherapies and other psychosocial treatments in conjunction with psychiatric management may also help address certain comorbid disorders or environmental or psychosocial stressors.

Antidepressant medications
- Tricyclic antidepressants (TCAs), selective serotonin reuptake inhibitors (SSRIs), and monoamine oxidase inhibitors (MAOIs) generally take 4 to 6 weeks to become effective for panic disorder.
- Because of their side effects and the need for dietary restrictions, MAOIs are generally reserved for patients who do not respond to other treatments.
- With all antidepressants, use doses approximately half of those given to depressed patients at the beginning of treatment because of possible hypersensitivity.
- Increase to a full therapeutic dose over subsequent days and weeks and as tolerated by the patient.

Benzodiazepines (for early symptom control)
- In combination with other treatment modalities, benzodiazepines are useful during initial treatment for more urgent relief of disabling anticipatory anxiety and panic attacks.
- Weigh the potential benefits of benzodiazepines against the following risks:
  - The patient may misattribute the entire treatment response to initial administration of the benzodiazepine and have difficulty with benzodiazepine discontinuation.
  - Anxiety relief may reduce motivation to engage in CBT.
  - Some patients experience withdrawal reactions upon discontinuation, even after relatively brief periods of benzodiazepine treatment.
- To counteract these risks, reassure the patient that definitive treatment takes a few weeks.
- To prevent development of high steady-state benzodiazepine levels and the risk of dependency, avoid unnecessarily high doses.

4. Length of Treatment

When determining length of treatment, consider the following:

- Successful treatment in the acute phase is indicated by markedly fewer and less intense panic attacks, less worry about panic attacks, and minimal or no phobic avoidance.
- With either CBT or antipanic medication, the acute phase of treatment lasts approximately 12 weeks.
- Some improvement is likely with either medication or CBT within 6 to 8 weeks (although full response may take longer).
- If there is no improvement within 6 to 8 weeks with a particular treatment, reevaluate the diagnosis and consider the need for a different treatment or the need for a combined treatment approach.
- If response to medication or CBT is not as expected, or if there are repeated relapses, evaluate for possible addition of a psychodynamic or other psychosocial intervention.
- After CBT treatment during the acute phase, decrease visit frequency and eventually discontinue treatment within several months.
- After 12 to 18 months, discontinuation of medication can be attempted with close follow-up.
- In case of relapse, resume the treatment that had proven effective.

B. Psychiatric Management

1. Evaluate particular symptoms.

▶ Promote patient perception that the psychiatrist accurately understands the patient's individual experience of panic.

▶ Be aware that a particular constellation of symptoms and other problems may influence treatment.

▶ Encourage the patient to self-monitor (e.g., by maintaining a daily diary) the frequency and nature of panic attacks plus the relationship between panic and internal and external stimuli.

2. Evaluate types and severity of functional impairment.

▶ Monitor anticipatory anxiety in addition to panic attacks.

▶ Assess the extent of phobic avoidance, which may determine the degree of impairment.

▶ Encourage the patient to define a desirable level of functioning.

3. Establish and maintain a therapeutic alliance.

Support the patient's efforts to confront phobic avoidance.

Assure the patient of therapist availability in case of emergencies to counteract patient's sensitivity to separations.

Be attuned and responsive to transference and countertransference phenomena.

4. Monitor the patient's psychiatric status.

Note that different elements of panic disorder often resolve at different times.

Continue to monitor the status of all presenting symptoms.

Monitor the success of the treatment plan on an ongoing basis.

Attend to the possibility of emergent depression.

Address any contributing comorbid psychiatric conditions.

5. Provide education.

Provide initial and ongoing education to the patient.
- Educate the patient about the disorder, its clinical course, and its complications.
- Emphasize that panic disorder is a real illness requiring support and treatment.
- Reassure the patient that panic attacks reflect real physiological events, but that the attacks themselves are not acutely dangerous or life threatening.

When appropriate, provide education to the family.
- Provide family members and significant others with information similar to that given to the patient.
- Help the family understand that attacks are terrifying to the patient and that panic disorder is debilitating if untreated.

6. Consider issues involved in working with other physicians.

Educate nonpsychiatric physicians who are also treating the patient.
- Recognize that a variety of general medical physicians may be involved because patients are often convinced that attacks are a manifestation of serious medical abnormalities.
- Educate other physicians as necessary about the ability of panic attacks to masquerade as many other general medical conditions.

Intervene as necessary to ensure that the patient continues to receive an appropriate level of medical care from the primary care physician and medical specialists.

7. Enhance treatment adherence.

Be aware that treatment (e.g., taking medication, confronting phobic stimuli) may initially increase anxiety and lead to nonadherence.

Conduct treatment in a supportive manner.

Discuss the patient's fears and provide reassurance, nonpunitive acceptance, and educational measures.

Consider enlisting the assistance of family members in improving the patient's adherence.

For persistent nonadherence, consider a psychodynamic treatment approach to address possible unconscious resistance.

8. Address early signs of relapse.

Respond to exacerbations that occur during treatment.
• Reassure the patient that fluctuations in symptoms can occur during treatment.
• Evaluate whether changes in the treatment plan are warranted.

Respond to relapses that occur after treatment ends.
Instruct patients that it is important to reinitiate treatment quickly to avoid the onset of complications such as phobic avoidance.

C. Treatment Interventions

1. Psychosocial Interventions

Cognitive behavior therapy
CBT may include the following components:
- Psychoeducation
  - Identify and name the patient's symptoms.
  - Provide a direct explanation of the basis for the symptoms.
  - Outline a plan for treatment.
- Continuous monitoring of panic attacks and anxious cognitions
- Daily anxiety-management techniques (e.g., abdominal breathing retraining) to reduce physiological reactivity
- Cognitive restructuring
  - Help the patient identify distorted thinking about sensations (e.g., overestimation of probability of negative consequence and other catastrophic thinking).
  - Encourage the patient to consider the evidence and think of alternative possible outcomes.
- Exposure to fear cues
  - Cues may be internal or environmental.
  - Direct the patient to identify a hierarchy of fear-evoking situations.
  - Encourage the patient to confront feared situations on a regular (usually daily) basis until the fear has attenuated.

Psychodynamic and other psychotherapies
- Psychodynamic and other psychotherapies may be the treatment of choice for some patients.
- The goal of psychodynamic psychotherapy is to elucidate and resolve conflicts and unconscious processes that may be causing or increasing vulnerability to the occurrence of panic symptoms.
- Use the therapeutic relationship to focus on unconscious symptom determinants.
- Place symptoms in the context of the patient's developmental history and current relationships and realities.

1. Psychosocial Interventions (continued)

Patient support groups
- Support groups may give patients the opportunity to recognize that their experiences with panic disorder are not unique and to share coping strategies.
- Such groups may complement other therapies but cannot substitute for effective treatment.

2. Pharmacotherapies

Selective serotonin reuptake inhibitors
- For many patients, SSRIs provide the most favorable balance of efficacy versus adverse effects.
- Response usually takes at least 4 weeks; for some patients, full response takes 8 to 12 weeks.
- Taper SSRIs (except for fluoxetine) over several weeks if discontinuing them after prolonged use.

Tricyclic antidepressants
- TCAs may be suboptimal in suicidal patients because overdose may be fatal.
- A common strategy is to start with 10 mg/day (of imipramine or equivalent) and titrate upward gradually (because of the possibility of initial stimulant response).
- Maintain an initial target dosage of 100 mg/day for 4 weeks; if no response or inadequate response, increase to a total of 300 mg/day as needed.
- Wait at least 6 weeks after initiation of TCA treatment (with at least 2 of those weeks at full dose) before deciding whether a TCA is effective.

Benzodiazepines
- Benzodiazepines may be used preferentially in situations in which very rapid control of symptoms is critical (e.g., the patient is about to quit school, lose a job, or require hospitalization).
- An effective dosage of alprazolam may be 1 to 2 mg/day, although many patients require 5 to 6 mg/day (in divided doses from two to four times per day); other benzodiazepines are effective at equivalent dosages.
- Even after 6 to 8 weeks of treatment, withdrawal symptoms and symptom rebound commonly occur when benzodiazepines are discontinued. Yet there is little dose escalation with long-term use.
- To discontinue, taper very slowly, probably over 2 to 4 months and at rates no greater than 10% of the dose per week.
- Benzodiazepine use is generally contraindicated for patients with a history of substance use disorder.

Monoamine oxidase inhibitors
- The commonly held belief that MAOIs are more potent antipanic agents than TCAs has never been convincingly proved.
- Although MAOIs are effective, they are generally reserved for patients who do not respond to other treatments. This is due to the risk of hypertensive crises, necessary dietary restrictions, and other side effects.

Other antidepressants
Limited data support the use of venlafaxine and nefazodone but not bupropion.

APPENDIX A. Advantages and Disadvantages of Treatment Modalities

Modality	Advantages	Disadvantages
Psychotherapies		
Panic-focused CBT	• Minimal side effects compared with pharmacotherapies • No risk of physiological dependency	• Patient must be willing to do "homework" (e.g., breathing exercises, recording of anxious cognitions) and confront feared situations • Lack of availability in some regions
Other psychotherapies (e.g., psychodynamic psychotherapy, family therapy)	• May be the treatment of choice for some patients (e.g., those with prominent personality disorder or psychological conflicts)	• Efficacy is less well studied compared with CBT
Pharmacotherapies		
SSRIs	• Ready availability • Fewer serious adverse side effects compared with TCAs and MAOIs • No potential for the physiological dependency associated with benzodiazepines	• Sexual side effects • Cost may be higher compared with other medication classes
TCAs	• Ready availability • Tolerated by most patients, although generally not as well as SSRIs, venlafaxine, or nefazodone • No potential for the physiological dependency associated with benzodiazepines	• Risks of cardiovascular and anticholinergic side effects (especially for the elderly or patients with general medical problems) • Suboptimal for suicidal patients because overdose may be fatal
Benzodiazepines	• Ready availability • Rapid control of symptoms	• Risk of tolerance, dependence, and withdrawal symptoms • In elderly, risk of confusion and falls
MAOIs	• Ready availability • No potential for the physiological dependency associated with benzodiazepines	• Risk of hypertensive crises • Dietary restrictions • Other adverse side effects • Suboptimal for suicidal patients because overdose may be fatal
Other antidepressants	• Ready availability • For some patients, a more tolerable side effect profile than other classes of antidepressants • No potential for the physiological dependency associated with benzodiazepines	• Limited data support the use of venlafaxine and nefazodone • There is general consensus that bupropion is not effective for panic symptoms

TREATING
EATING DISORDERS
A Quick Reference Guide

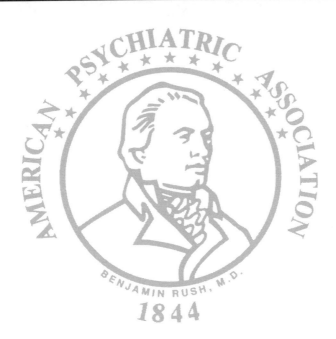

Based on *Practice Guideline for the Treatment of Patients With Eating Disorders,* Second Edition, originally published in January 2000. A guideline watch, summarizing significant developments in the scientific literature since publication of this guideline, may be available in the Psychiatric Practice section of the APA web site at www.psych.org.

OUTLINE

A. Initial Assessment and Diagnosis

The psychiatrist will consider the following areas of assessment:

1. Diagnostic Criteria

> Review DSM-IV-TR criteria for anorexia nervosa (DSM-IV-TR, p. 589) and bulimia nervosa (DSM-IV-TR, p. 594).

2. General Medical Status

> Conduct a physical examination with particular attention to the following:
> - Vital signs
> - Weight
> - Physical and sexual growth and development
> - Cardiovascular system and evidence of dehydration
> - Lanugo
> - Salivary gland enlargement
> - Russell's sign (scarring on dorsum of hand)

> Review dental examination results.

> Conduct laboratory analyses, as indicated.
> For laboratory assessments and their patient indications, refer to Appendix A in this guide (p. 158).

3. Potential for Dangerousness

Determine danger to self.
Assess current suicidal ideation, history of suicidal ideation, suicide attempts, and self-mutilation.

Determine access to means for suicide.

4. Eating Disorder Symptoms and Behaviors

Obtain a detailed report of a single day.

Observe the patient during a meal.

Assess related psychological symptoms—for example, obsessional thoughts related to weight, shape, and eating.

Determine the patient's insight into the presence of the disorder and the patient's motivation for change.

Explore the patient's understanding of how the illness developed and the effects of interpersonal problems on onset.

Identify those stressors that exacerbate the symptoms of the eating disorder.

Consider the use of formal measures—for example, scales for assessments of symptoms such as binge frequency.

5. Other Psychiatric Symptoms and Behaviors

Assess the following:
- Mood symptoms and disorders
- Anxiety symptoms and disorders
- Obsessions/compulsions
- Substance abuse
- Shoplifting; other impulsive behaviors
- Personality disturbances

6. Psychiatric History

Assess previous episodes and previous treatment response.

7. Developmental and Psychosocial History

Assess the following:
- Psychological, sexual, or physical abuse
- Sexual history
- Psychodynamic and interpersonal conflicts relevant to understanding and treating the patient's eating disorder

8. Family Issues

Assess the following:
- Family history of eating disorders, other psychiatric disorders, obesity
- Family reactions to disorder; attitudes toward eating, exercise, and appearance
- Burden of illness on family
- Family dynamics: guilt, blame

B. Psychiatric Management

Throughout the formulation of a treatment plan and the subsequent course of treatment, the following principles of psychiatric management should be kept in mind:

Establish and maintain a therapeutic alliance.
- Adapt and modify therapeutic strategies as the disorder and the therapeutic alliance change over time.
- Build the alliance by acknowledging the patient's difficulties in gaining weight.
- Be aware of countertransference reactions.
- Set clear boundaries.

Provide and/or coordinate care and collaborate with other clinicians.
- Collaborate with providers of nutritional counseling, family work, and various psychotherapeutic programs (e.g., individual, group, cognitive/behavioral).
- Consult with other physician specialists and dentists.
- Educate and supervise inexperienced staff.

Monitor eating disorder symptoms and behaviors.

Ensure that the patient's general medical status is monitored.
- Weight and vital signs
- Food and fluid intake and output
- Periodic physical examinations, with special attention to signs of edema and fluid overload
- Urine specific gravity
- Minerals and electrolytes

Monitor the patient's psychiatric status, safety, and comorbid conditions.

C. Treatment Goals and Ongoing Assessment

Following diagnosis, set treatment goals, assess ongoing progress, and adjust goals accordingly. Other treatment goals may be identified, depending on the patient's needs and condition.

1. Anorexia Nervosa

➤ *Restore healthy weight.*

➤ Treat physical complications.

➤ Enhance the patient's motivation to cooperate and participate in treatment.

➤ Provide education about healthy nutrition and eating patterns.

➤ Correct core maladaptive thoughts and attitudes.

➤ Treat associated psychiatric conditions, including defects in mood regulation, self-esteem, and behavior.

➤ Enlist family support and provide family counseling and therapy where appropriate.

➤ Prevent relapse.

2. Bulimia Nervosa

> *Reduce binge eating and purging behaviors.*

> Improve attitudes related to eating disorders.

> Minimize food restrictions.

> Encourage healthy but not excessive exercise.

> Treat comorbid conditions.

> **Address underlying themes:**
> - Developmental issues
> - Identity formation
> - Body image concerns
> - Self-esteem in areas outside weight and shape
> - Difficulties with sexual issues and aggression
> - Affect regulation
> - Gender role expectations
> - Family dysfunction
> - Coping styles

D. Treatment

1. Anorexia Nervosa
a. *Treatment Setting*

Weight and cardiac status are the most important physical parameters in determining choice of setting. The strategy is to hospitalize *before* a patient becomes medically unstable.

Medical indications for inpatient hospitalization

Adults
- Weight < 75% of standard
- Heart rate < 40 bpm
- Blood pressure < 90/60 mm Hg
- Glucose < 60 mg/dL
- Potassium < 3 meq/L
- Electrolyte imbalance
- Temperature < 97.0°F
- Dehydration
- Hepatic, renal, or cardiovascular organ compromise requiring acute treatment

Children and Adolescents
- Weight < 75% of standard or acute weight decline with food refusal
- Heart rate 40–49 bpm
- Orthostatic hypotension (with an increase in pulse of > 20 bpm or a drop in blood pressure of > 10–20 mm Hg/minute from supine to standing
- Blood pressure < 80/50 mm Hg
- Hypokalemia or hypophosphatemia

Other factors influencing decision about inpatient hospitalization
- Suicidal intent and plan
- Poor motivation to recover
- Preoccupation with ego-syntonic thoughts
- Uncooperative with treatment or cooperative only in highly structured settings
- Any existing psychiatric disorder that would require hospitalization
- Need for supervision during and after all meals and in bathrooms
- Presence of additional stressors interfering with ability to eat (e.g., intercurrent viral illnesses)
- Knowledge of weight at which instability is likely to occur

1. Anorexia Nervosa
a. *Treatment Setting* (continued)

Psychiatric versus general hospitalization
Consider the following:
• General medical status of the patient
• Skills and abilities of local care providers
• Availability of suitable intensive outpatient, partial and day hospitalization, and aftercare programs

Patient factors influencing decision about placement in a residential treatment center
• Medical stability to the extent that intravenous fluids, nasogastric tube feedings, or multiple daily laboratory tests are not needed
• Weight < 85% of standard
• Poor to fair motivation to recover
• Preoccupation with ego-syntonic maladaptive thoughts about 4 to 6 hours a day; cooperative with highly structured treatment
• Need for supervision at all meals to prevent restrictive eating
• Pronounced role impairment and inability to eat and gain weight by self
• Need for structure to prevent compulsive exercising
• Severe family conflict or problems; absence of family, adequate support system, or both

Patient factors influencing decision about partial hospitalization (full-day outpatient care)
• Partial motivation to recover
• Preoccupation with ego-syntonic maladaptive thoughts at least 3 hours a day
• Need for structure to gain weight
• Need for structure to prevent compulsive exercising
• Presence of comorbid psychiatric conditions requiring intensive treatment

1. Anorexia Nervosa
b. Nutritional Rehabilitation

Phase 1: Refeeding and weight gain
- Establish the target weight and rates of weight gain: a healthy goal weight is the weight at which normal menstruation and ovulation are restored or, in premenarchal girls, the weight at which normal physical and sexual development resumes.
- Usually start intake at 30 to 40 kcal/kg per day (approximately 1000 to 1600 kcal/day); intake may be increased to as high as 70 to 100 kcal/kg per day.
- Nasogastric feeding is reserved for the rare patients who are extremely unable to recognize their illness, accept the need for treatment, or tolerate guilt accompanying active eating even when performed to sustain life.
- Add vitamin and mineral supplements; for example, phosphorus supplementation may be particularly useful to prevent serum hypophosphatemia.
- Help the patient limit physical activity and caloric expenditure according to food intake and fitness requirements.
- Monitor vital signs; food and fluid intake/output; electrolytes; signs of fluid overload (e.g., presence of edema, rapid weight gain, congestive heart failure); and gastrointestinal symptoms, particularly constipation and bloating. Provide cardiac monitoring, especially at night, for children and adolescents who are severely malnourished.

Phase 2: Weight maintenance
- Once the desired weight is achieved, calculate ongoing caloric intake based on weight and activity. For children and adolescents, intake levels at 40 to 60 kcal/day are often needed for growth and maturation.
- Help the patient deal with concerns about weight gain and body image changes.
- Educate about the risks of eating disorders.
- Provide ongoing support to the patient and the family.

1. Anorexia Nervosa
c. Psychosocial Treatments

Establishing and maintaining a psychotherapeutically informed relationship with the patient is important and beneficial. Psychosocial interventions need to be informed by an understanding of psychodynamic conflicts, cognitive development, psychological defenses, and the complexity of family relationships, as well as the presence of other psychiatric disorders. Formal psychotherapy may be helpful after weight gain has started.

Individual psychotherapy
Usually required for at least 1 year. May take 5 to 6 years because of the enduring nature of the illness and the need for support during recovery.

Family and couples therapy
Useful when problems in familial relationships are contributing to the maintenance of the disorder.

Group psychotherapy
Care must be taken to help patients avoid competition to be thinnest or sickest and to deal with patient demoralization from observation of the difficult, chronic course of the illness.

1. Anorexia Nervosa
d. Medications

Psychotropic medications should not be relied on as the sole or primary treatment of anorexia nervosa. Decisions concerning use of medications are often deferred until weight has been restored because many symptoms (including depression) diminish considerably when weight is gained.

After weight restoration
- Antidepressants for persistent depression or anxiety
- Selective serotonin reuptake inhibitors (SSRIs) for obsessive-compulsive symptoms

Additional considerations
- Malnourished, depressed patients are more prone to side effects.
- Bupropion should be avoided in patients with eating disorders.
- Tricyclic antidepressants (TCAs) should be avoided in underweight patients and those at risk for suicide.
- Cardiovascular consultation may be helpful if there is concern about the potential cardiovascular effects of a medication.

2. Bulimia Nervosa
a. Treatment Setting

Most patients with uncomplicated bulimia nervosa do not require hospitalization.

Factors supporting inpatient hospitalization
- Severe, disabling symptoms that have not responded to outpatient treatment
- Serious concurrent general medical problems (e.g., metabolic abnormalities, hematemesis, vital sign changes, or the appearance of uncontrolled vomiting)
- Suicidality
- Severe concurrent alcohol or drug abuse

2. Bulimia Nervosa
b. Nutritional Rehabilitation

Weight restoration is usually not a primary focus of treatment for bulimia nervosa because patients are not severely underweight.

Nutritional counseling is helpful for the following:
- Establishing a pattern of regular, nonbinge meals
- Increasing the variety of foods eaten
- Correcting nutritional deficiencies
- Minimizing food restriction
- Encouraging healthy but not excessive exercise patterns

2. Bulimia Nervosa
c. Psychosocial Treatments

Psychosocial interventions should be informed by a comprehensive evaluation of the patient, including cognitive and psychological development, psychodynamic issues, cognitive style, comorbid psychopathology, patient preferences, and family situation. Controlled studies have been short-term, but long-term psychotherapy may be needed for patients with concurrent anorexia nervosa or severe personality disorders.

Cognitive behavior therapy
- Effective as a short-term intervention when specifically directed at eating disorder symptoms and underlying maladaptive cognitions
- Useful in reducing binge-eating symptoms and improving attitudes about shape, weight, and restrictive dieting

Interpersonal psychotherapy, psychodynamically oriented and psychoanalytic approaches, and behavior techniques (e.g., planned meals, self-monitoring) may also be helpful.

Group psychotherapy
- Can help the patient with shame about the disorder
- Provides peer-based feedback and support
- Is more useful if dietary counseling and management are included in the program

Family and marital therapy
Should be considered especially for adolescents who live with parents, for older patients with ongoing conflicted interaction with parents, or for patients with marital discord

2. Bulimia Nervosa
d. Medications

Indications
- To reduce frequency of disturbed eating behaviors (binge eating and vomiting)
- To prevent relapse—most clinicians recommend continuation for 6 months to 1 year
- To reduce associated symptoms (e.g., depression, anxiety, obsessions, symptoms related to impulse control)

Considerations
- Various antidepressants may have to be tried sequentially to achieve optimum effect.
- If no response, the clinician should assess whether the patient has taken medication shortly before vomiting; serum levels may be helpful.
- A combination of psychotherapy and medication may be superior to either alone.

Classes
- SSRIs are considered safest and are helpful for depression, anxiety, obsessions, and certain impulse disorder symptoms and for patients with a suboptimal response to appropriate psychosocial therapy. Doses may need to be higher than those used to treat depression (e.g., 60 to 80 mg of fluoxetine).
- Antidepressant medications from a variety of other classes can reduce the symptoms of binge eating and purging and may help prevent relapse.

Caveats
- TCAs should be used with caution for patients at high risk of suicide.
- Monoamine oxidase inhibitors (MAOIs) should be avoided for patients with chaotic binge eating and purging.
- Bupropion should be avoided in patients with bulimia because of increased seizure risk.

Side effects and toxicity
- SSRIs: insomnia, nausea, asthenia, sexual side effects.
- TCAs: sedation, constipation, dry mouth, weight gain.
- For patients who need mood stabilizers, lithium carbonate may be particularly problematic, because levels can shift markedly with rapid volume changes. Both lithium and valproic acid are associated with undesirable weight gain.

APPENDIX A. Laboratory Assessments for Patients With Eating Disorders

Assessment	Condition

Basic analyses
Blood chemistry studies
  Serum electrolyte level
  Blood urea nitrogen (BUN) level
  Creatinine level
  Thyroid function test
Complete blood count (CBC)
Urinalysis
	• Consider for all patients with eating disorders

Additional analyses
Blood chemistry studies
  Calcium level
  Magnesium level
  Phosphorus level
  Liver function tests
Electrocardiogram
	• Consider for malnourished and severely symptomatic patients

Osteopenia and osteoporosis assessments Dual-energy X-ray absorptiometry (DEXA) Estradiol level Testosterone level in males	• Consider for patients underweight more than 6 months
Nonroutine assessments	• Consider only for specific indications
Serum amylase level	• Possible indicator of persistent or recurrent vomiting
Luteinizing hormone (LH) and follicle-stimulating hormone (FSH) levels	• For persistent amenorrhea at normal weight
Brain magnetic resonance imaging (MRI) and computed tomography (CT)	• For ventricular enlargement correlated with degree of malnutrition
Stool	• Occult blood loss; suspected surreptitious laxative abuse

TREATING BORDERLINE PERSONALITY DISORDER

A Quick Reference Guide

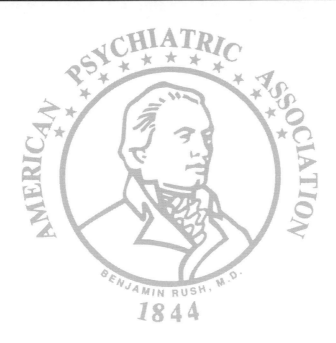

Based on *Practice Guideline for the Treatment of Patients With Borderline Personality Disorder,* originally published in October 2001. A guideline watch, summarizing significant developments in the scientific literature since publication of this guideline, may be available in the Psychiatric Practice section of the APA web site at www.psych.org.

OUTLINE

A. Initial Presentation

1. Initial Assessment to Determine Treatment Setting

Consider *partial hospitalization* (or brief inpatient hospitalization if partial hospitalization is not available) if any of the following are present:
- Dangerous impulsive behavior that cannot be managed with outpatient treatment
- Deteriorating clinical picture related to nonadherence to outpatient treatment
- Complex comorbidity that requires more intensive clinical assessment of treatment response
- Symptoms that are unresponsive to outpatient treatment and that are of sufficient severity to interfere with work, family life, or other significant domains of functioning

Consider *brief inpatient hospitalization* if any of the following are present:
- Imminent danger to others
- Loss of control of suicidal impulses or serious suicide attempt
- Transient psychotic episode associated with loss of impulse control, impaired judgment, or both
- Symptoms that are unresponsive to outpatient treatment and partial hospitalization and that are of sufficient severity to interfere with work, family life, or other significant domains of functioning

1. Initial Assessment to Determine Treatment Setting *(continued)*

→ **Consider *extended inpatient hospitalization* if any of the following are present:**
- Persistent, severe suicidality or self-destructiveness
- Nonadherence to outpatient or partial hospital treatment
- Comorbid refractory axis I disorder (e.g., eating disorder, mood disorder) that is potentially life threatening
- Comorbid substance dependence or abuse that is severe and unresponsive to outpatient treatment or partial hospitalization
- Continued risk of assaultive behavior toward others despite brief hospitalization
- Symptoms of sufficient severity to interfere with functioning and work or family life and that are unresponsive to outpatient treatment and partial hospitalization or brief hospitalization

2. Comprehensive Evaluation

→ **Follow initial assessment with a more comprehensive evaluation that considers a wide range of domains and issues, including**
- Presence of comorbid disorders
- Degree and types of functional impairment
- Intrapsychic conflicts and defenses
- Developmental progress and arrests
- Adaptive and maladaptive coping styles
- Psychosocial stressors and strengths in the face of stressors

(See also APA's *Practice Guideline for Psychiatric Evaluation of Adults*.)

→ **Consider additional sources of information (e.g., medical records, informants who know the patient well) in the assessment process because of patient denial and the ego-syntonicity of personality traits and behaviors.**

3. Treatment Framework

Establish a clear treatment framework (e.g., a treatment contract) with explicit agreements about the following:
- Goals of treatment sessions (e.g., symptom reduction, personal growth, improvement in functioning)
- When, where, and with what frequency sessions will be held
- A plan for crises
- Clarification of the clinician's after-hours availability
- Fees, billing, and payment

B. Psychiatric Management

The primary treatment for borderline personality disorder is psychotherapy, which may be complemented by symptom-targeted pharmacotherapy. Throughout the course of treatment, it is important to provide psychiatric management as follows:

Respond to crises and monitor the patient's safety.
- Evaluate self-injurious or suicidal ideas.
- Assess the potential dangerousness of behaviors, the patient's motivations, and the extent to which the patient can manage his or her safety without external interventions.
- Reformulate the treatment plan as appropriate.
- Consider hospitalization if the patient's safety is judged to be at serious risk.

B. Psychiatric Management *(continued)*

Establish and maintain a therapeutic framework and alliance.
- Recognize that patients with borderline personality disorder have difficulty developing and sustaining trusting relationships.
- Ascertain that the patient agrees with and explicitly accepts the treatment plan.
- Establish and reinforce an understanding about respective roles and responsibilities regarding the attainment of treatment goals.
- Encourage patients to be actively engaged in the treatment, both in their tasks (e.g., monitoring medication effects or noting and reflecting on their feelings) and in the relationship (e.g., disclosing reactions to or wishes toward the clinician).
- Focus attention on whether the patient understands and accepts what the psychiatrist says, and whether the patient feels understood and accepted.

Collaborate with the patient in solving practical problems, giving advice and guidance when needed.

Provide education about borderline personality disorder and its treatment.
- Familiarize the patient with the diagnosis, including its expected course, responsiveness to treatment, and, when appropriate, known pathogenic factors.
- Provide ongoing education about self-care (e.g., safe sex, potential legal problems, sleep, and diet) if appropriate.
- Consider psychoeducation for families or others who live with patients.

Coordinate treatment provided by multiple clinicians.
- Establish clear role definitions, plans for crisis management, and regular communication among the clinicians.
- Determine which clinician is assuming primary overall responsibility. This clinician will
  - serve as a gatekeeper for the appropriate level of care,
  - oversee family involvement,
  - lead decision making regarding which treatment modalities are useful or should be changed or discontinued,
  - help assess the impact of medications, and
  - monitor the patient's safety.

Monitor and reassess the patient's clinical status and treatment plan.
- Be alert for declines in function.
  - Regressive phenomena may arise if the patient believes he or she no longer needs to be as responsible for self-care.
  - Declines in function are likely to occur during reductions in the intensity or amount of support.
  - If declines during exploratory therapy are sustained, consider shifting treatment focus from exploration to other psychotherapeutic and educational strategies.
- Critically examine apparent medication "breakthroughs" (i.e., sustained return of symptoms that had remitted apparently because of medications).
  - Consider whether breakthroughs are transitory, reactive moods in response to an interpersonal crisis.
  - Avoid frequent medication changes in pursuit of improving transient mood states.
- Consider introducing changes in treatment if the patient fails to show improvement in targeted goals by 6 to 12 months.
- Consider consultation if the patient continues to do poorly after treatment is modified.

B. Psychiatric Management *(continued)*

Periodically consider arranging for a consultation if there is no improvement (e.g., less distress, more adaptive behaviors, greater trust) during treatment.

A low threshold for seeking consultation should occur in the presence of any of the following:
- High frequency of countertransference reactions and medicolegal liability complications
- High frequency of complicated multiclinician, multimodality treatments
- High level of inference, subjectivity, and life-and-death significance involved in clinical judgments

Be aware of and manage potential splitting and boundary problems.
- If splitting threatens continuation of the treatment, consider altering treatment (e.g., increasing support, seeking consultation).
- To avoid splitting within the treatment team, facilitate communication among team members.
- Be explicit in establishing "boundaries" around the treatment relationship and task.
- Maintain consistency with agreed-on boundaries.
- Be aware that it is the therapist's responsibility to monitor and sustain the treatment boundaries.
- In the event of a boundary crossing,
  - explore the meaning of the boundary crossing;
  - restate expectations about the boundary and rationale; and
  - if the boundary crossing continues, employ limit setting.
- Making exceptions to the usual treatment boundaries may signal the need for consultation or supervision.
- Sexual interaction with a patient is always unethical; if it occurs, the patient should be immediately referred to another therapist. The therapist involved in the boundary violation should seek consultation or personal psychotherapy.

C. Principles of Treatment Selection

1. Type of Treatment

- Most patients will need extended psychotherapy to attain and maintain lasting improvement in their personality, interpersonal problems, and overall functioning.
- Pharmacotherapy often has an important adjunctive role, especially for diminution of symptoms such as affective instability, impulsivity, psychotic-like symptoms, and self-destructive behavior.
- Many patients will benefit most from a combination of psychotherapy and pharmacotherapy.

2. Flexibility and Comprehensiveness of the Treatment Plan

- Treatment planning should address borderline personality disorder as well as comorbid axis I and axis II disorders, with priority established according to risk or predominant symptomatology.
- The treatment plan must be flexible, adapted to the needs of the individual patient.
- The plan also must respond to the changing characteristics of the patient over time.

3. Role of Patient Preference

- Discuss the range of treatments available for the patient's condition and what the psychiatrist recommends.
- Elicit the patient's views and modify the plan to the extent feasible to take these views and preferences into account.

4. Single Versus Multiple Clinicians

- Both are viable approaches.
- Treatment by multiple clinicians has potential advantages but may become fragmented.
- Good collaboration of the treatment team and clarity about roles and responsibility are essential.
- The effectiveness of single versus multiple clinicians should be monitored over time and changed if the patient is not improving.

D. Specific Treatment Strategies

1. Individual Psychotherapeutic Approaches

Two psychotherapeutic approaches have been shown to have efficacy: psychoanalytic/psychodynamic therapies and dialectical behavior therapy. The key features shared by these approaches suggest that the following can help guide the psychiatrist treating a patient with borderline personality disorder, regardless of the specific type of therapy used:

Expect treatment to be long-term.
Substantial improvement may not occur until at least 1 year of treatment, and many patients require longer treatment.

Create a hierarchy of priorities to be considered in the treatment (e.g., first focus on suicidal behavior).
For examples, see Figure 1 in APA's *Practice Guideline for the Treatment of Patients With Borderline Personality Disorder.*

Monitor self-destructive and suicidal behaviors.

Build a strong therapeutic alliance that includes empathic validation of the patient's suffering and experience.

Help the patient take appropriate responsibility for his or her actions.
• Minimize self-blame for past abuse.
• Encourage responsibility for avoiding current self-destructive patterns.
• Focus interventions more on the here and now than on the distant past.

Use a flexible strategy, depending on the current situation.
• When appropriate, offer interpretations to help develop insight.
• At other times, it may be more therapeutic to provide validation, empathy, and advice.

Appropriately manage intense feelings engendered in both the patient and the therapist.
• Consider the use of professional supervision and consultation.
• Also consider personal psychotherapy.

Promote reflection rather than impulsive action.
• Promote self-observation to generate a greater understanding of how behaviors may originate from internal motivations and affect states.
• Encourage thinking through the consequences of actions.

Diminish splitting.
• Help the patient integrate positive and negative aspects of self and others.
• Encourage recognition that perceptions are representations rather than how things are.

Set limits on the patient's self-destructive behaviors and, if necessary, convey the limitations of the therapist's capacities (e.g., spell out minimal conditions necessary for therapy to be viable).

2. Other Forms of Psychotherapy

Group therapy may be helpful but offers no clear advantage over individual therapy.
- Group therapy is usually used in combination with individual therapy.
- Relatively homogeneous groups are recommended. Exclude from groups patients with antisocial personality disorder, untreated substance abuse, or psychosis.

Couples therapy may be a useful adjunctive modality but is not recommended as the only form of treatment for patients with borderline personality disorder.

Family therapy is most helpful when the patient has significant involvement with family.
- Whether to work with the family should depend on family pathology, strengths, and weaknesses.
- Family therapy is not recommended as the only form of treatment for patients with borderline personality disorder.

3. Pharmacotherapy and Other Somatic Treatments

Principles for choosing specific medications include the following:
- Treatment is symptom specific, directed at particular behavioral dimensions.
- Affective dysregulation and impulsivity/aggression are risk factors for suicidal behavior, self-injury, and assaultiveness and are given high priority in selecting pharmacological agents.
- Medication targets both acute symptoms (e.g., anger treated with dopamine-blocking agents) and chronic vulnerabilities (e.g., temperamental impulsivity treated with serotonergic agents).

Symptoms to be targeted

Affective dysregulation symptoms (see Figure 1, p. 172)

Treat initially with a selective serotonin reuptake inhibitor (SSRI). A reasonable trial is at least 12 weeks.

- Be cautious about discontinuing successful treatment, especially if the patient has failed to respond to prior medication trials.
- If response is suboptimal, switch to a different SSRI or a related antidepressant.
- Consider adding a benzodiazepine (especially clonazepam) when affective dysregulation presents as anxiety.
- For disinhibited anger coexisting with other affective symptoms, SSRIs are the treatment of choice.
- For severe behavioral dyscontrol, consider adding low-dose neuroleptics.
- Monoamine oxidase inhibitors (MAOIs) are effective but are not a first-line treatment because of the risk of serious side effects and concerns about nonadherence with dietary restrictions.
- Mood stabilizers (lithium, valproate, carbamazepine) are also a second-line treatment (or augmentation treatment).
- Consider electroconvulsive therapy (ECT) for comorbid severe axis I depression refractory to pharmacotherapy.

FIGURE 1. Psychopharmacological Treatment of Affective Dysregulation Symptoms in Patients With Borderline Personality Disorder

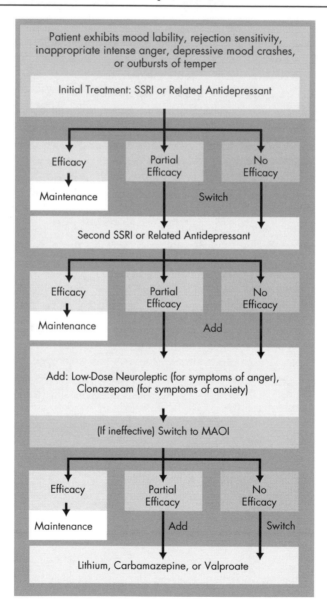

3. Pharmacotherapy and Other Somatic Treatments

Symptoms to be targeted *(continued)*

Impulsive-behavioral symptoms (see Figure 2, p. 174)

SSRIs are the treatment of choice.
- If a serious threat to the patient's safety is present, consider adding a low-dose neuroleptic to the SSRI. Onset of action is often within hours.
- If an SSRI is ineffective, consider another SSRI or another class of antidepressant.
- If the patient shows partial response to an SSRI, adding lithium may enhance the effectiveness of the SSRI.
- If an SSRI is ineffective, switching to an MAOI may be considered after an appropriate drug washout period.
- Consider valproate, carbamazepine, and atypical neuroleptics. There is widespread use of these agents despite limited data.
- Clozapine may be warranted after other treatments have failed.

Cognitive-perceptual symptoms (see Figure 3, p. 175)

- Low-dose neuroleptics are the treatment of choice for psychotic-like symptoms.
- Neuroleptics may also improve depressed mood, impulsivity, and anger-hostility.
- Neuroleptics are most effective when cognitive-perceptual symptoms are primary.
- If response is suboptimal in 4 to 6 weeks, increase dose to the range used for axis I disorders.
- Clozapine may be useful for patients with severe, refractory psychotic-like symptoms.

FIGURE 2. Psychopharmacological Treatment of Impulsive-Behavioral Dyscontrol Symptoms in Patients With Borderline Personality Disorder

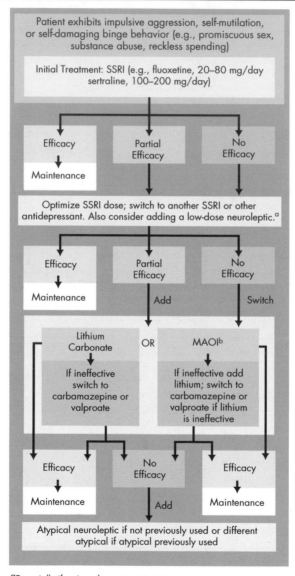

[a]Especially if serious threat to patient is present.

[b]SSRI treatment must be discontinued and followed with an adequate washout period before initiating treatment with an MAOI.

FIGURE 3. **Psychopharmacological Treatment of Cognitive-Perceptual Symptoms in Patients With Borderline Personality Disorder**

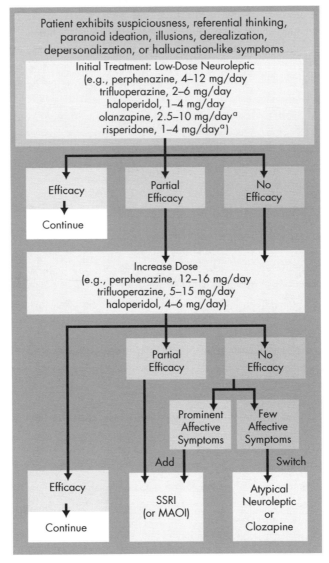

[a]The generally favorable side effect profiles of the newer atypical neuroleptic medications compared with those of conventional neuroleptics underscore the need for careful empirical trials of these newer medications in the treatment of patients with borderline personality disorder.

E. Special Features Influencing Treatment

Address comorbidity with axis I and other axis II disorders.
• For guidance, refer to other APA practice guidelines.
• Comorbid depression, often with atypical features, is particularly common.

Treat problematic substance use.
• Substance abuse often leads to less favorable outcomes, including increased risk of suicide or accidents.
• Substance abuse may lower threshold for other self-destructive behavior.
• Vigorous treatment is essential.

Address violent behavior and antisocial traits.
• For mild antisocial behavior, provide psychotherapy, psychoeducation, or both to help the patient understand the advantages of socially appropriate alternatives.
• For more severe antisocial behavior, consider residential treatment, mood stabilizers, or SSRIs.
• If antisocial traits predominate or threat of violence is imminent, psychotherapy may prove ineffective. If violence is threatened or imminent, hospitalization may be indicated and potential victims may need to be warned.

Address chronic self-destructive behavior.
• Limit setting is often necessary—consider a hierarchy of priorities (see Figure 1 of APA's *Practice Guideline for the Treatment of Patients With Borderline Personality Disorder*).
• Target behaviors that are destructive to the patient, the family, the therapist, or the therapy.
• If the patient is out of control, consider a more intensive treatment setting.

Address trauma and posttraumatic stress disorder (PTSD).
- It is important to recognize any existing trauma history.
- Recognize trauma transference issues (e.g., expectation that the therapist will be malevolent).
- Working through trauma is best done at a later phase of treatment; it involves exposure to memories, managing affect, and cognitive restructuring.
- Recognize that patients may be at increased risk of further trauma and revictimization.
- Group support and therapy can be helpful.
- Be aware of and treat PTSD-like symptoms if present.
- Clarify the patient's lack of responsibility for past trauma if appropriate and the importance of taking responsibility for present life circumstances.

Address dissociative features.
- Explore dissociative symptoms and their triggers.
- Teach the patient how to access and control dissociation.
- Facilitate integration of dissociative identities.
- Provide positive reinforcement for integrated functioning.

Address psychosocial stressors.
- Stressors, particularly of an interpersonal nature, may exacerbate symptoms.
- Limits of the therapeutic relationship may stimulate anxiety-driven reactions.

Consider gender, age, and cultural factors.
- Borderline personality disorder may be missed in males, who may be misdiagnosed as antisocial or narcissistic.
- Treatment of pregnant and nursing women raises special considerations regarding the use of psychotropic medications.
- Cultural factors may hamper accurate assessment. Cultural bias in assessment of sexual behavior, emotional expression, and impulsivity should be avoided.
- Diagnoses in adolescents should be made with care because personality is still developing.

F. Risk Management Issues

1. General Considerations

- Collaborate and communicate with other treating clinicians.
- Provide careful and adequate documentation, including assessment of risk, communication with other clinicians, the decision-making process, and the rationale for the treatment approach.
- Attend to problems in the transference and countertransference and be alert for splitting.
- Consider consultation with a colleague for unusually high-risk patients, when a patient is not improving, or when the best treatment approach is unclear.
- Follow standard guidelines for terminating treatment.
- Consider providing psychoeducation about the disorder (e.g., risks of the disorder and uncertainties of treatment outcome).
- Assess the risk of suicide; the potential for angry, impulsive, or violent behavior; and the potential for boundary violations.

2. Suicide

- Monitor the patient carefully for suicide risk and document these assessments.
- Actively treat comorbid axis I disorders, with particular attention to those that may contribute to or increase the risk of suicide.
- Take suicide threats seriously and address them with the patient.
- Consider consultation and/or hospitalization.
- In the absence of acute risk, address chronic suicidality in the therapy.
- Consider involving the family when the patient is either chronically or acutely suicidal.
- Do not allow a "suicide contract" to substitute for a careful and thorough clinical evaluation of the patient's suicidality.

3. Anger, Impulsivity, and Violence

- Monitor the patient carefully for impulsive or violent behavior.
- Address abandonment/rejection issues, anger, and impulsivity in the treatment, because they may be triggers of violence.
- Arrange for adequate coverage when away; carefully communicate plans for coverage to the patient and document the coverage.
- If threats toward others or threatening behavior is present, action may be necessary to protect self or others.

4. Potential Boundary Violations

- Monitor carefully and explore countertransference feelings toward the patient.
- Be alert to deviations from the usual way of practicing (e.g., appointments at unusual hours), which may be signs of countertransference problems.
- Avoid boundary violations such as the development of a personal friendship outside the professional situation or a sexual relationship with the patient.
- Get a consultation if there are striking deviations from the usual manner of practice.

ASSESSING AND TREATING
SUICIDAL BEHAVIORS
A Quick Reference Guide

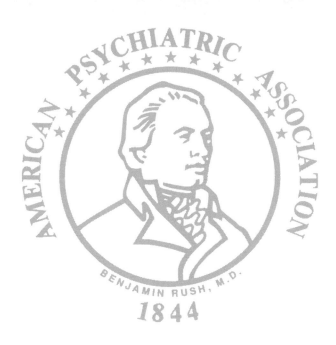

Based on *Practice Guideline for the Assessment and Treatment of Patients With Suicidal Behaviors*, originally published in November 2003. A guideline watch, summarizing significant developments in the scientific literature since publication of this guideline, may be available in the Psychiatric Practice section of the APA web site at www.psych.org.

OUTLINE

A. Assessment of Patients With Suicidal Behaviors

Refer to Table 1, p. 185, for circumstances in which suicide assessment may be indicated.

1. Conduct a thorough psychiatric evaluation.

Identify psychiatric signs and symptoms.
- Determine the presence or absence of signs and symptoms associated with specific psychiatric diagnoses.
- Identify specific psychiatric symptoms that may influence suicide risk, including aggression, violence toward others, impulsiveness, hopelessness, agitation, psychic anxiety, anhedonia, global insomnia, and panic attacks.

Assess past suicidal behavior, including intent of self-injurious acts.
- For each attempt, obtain details about the precipitants, timing, intent, consequences, and medical severity.
- Ascertain if alcohol and drugs were consumed before the attempt.
- Delineate interpersonal aspects of the attempt in order to understand issues that culminated in the attempt (e.g., persons present at the time of the attempt or to whom the attempt was communicated).
- Determine the patient's thoughts about the attempt (e.g., perception of potential for lethality, ambivalence toward living, visualization of death, degree of premeditation, persistence of suicidal ideation, and reaction to the attempt).

Review past treatment history and treatment relationships.
- Review psychiatric history (e.g., previous and comorbid diagnoses, prior hospitalizations and other treatment, past suicidal ideation).
- Review history of medical treatment (e.g., identify medically serious suicide attempts and past or current medical diagnoses).
- Gauge the strength and stability of current and past therapeutic relationships.

1. Conduct a thorough psychiatric evaluation *(continued).*

Identify family history of suicide, mental illness, and dysfunction.
- Inquire about family history of suicide and suicide attempts and psychiatric hospitalizations or mental illness, including substance use disorders.
- Determine the circumstances of suicides in first-degree relatives, including the patient's involvement and the patient's and relative's ages at the time.
- Determine childhood and current family milieu, including history of family conflict or separation, parental legal trouble, family substance use, domestic violence, and physical and/or sexual abuse.

Identify current psychosocial situation and nature of crisis.
Consider acute psychosocial crises or chronic psychosocial stressors that may augment suicide risk (e.g., financial or legal difficulties; interpersonal conflicts or losses; stressors in gay, lesbian, or bisexual youths; housing problems; job loss; educational failure).

Appreciate psychological strengths and vulnerabilities of the individual patient.
Consider how coping skills, personality traits, thinking style, and developmental and psychological needs may affect the patients' suicide risk and the formulation of the treatment plan.

TABLE 1. Circumstances in Which a Suicide Assessment May Be Indicated Clinically

- Emergency department or crisis evaluation
- Intake evaluation (on either an inpatient or an outpatient basis)
- Before a change in observation status or treatment setting (e.g., discontinuation of one-to-one observation, discharge from inpatient setting)
- Abrupt change in clinical presentation (either precipitous worsening or sudden, dramatic improvement)
- Lack of improvement or gradual worsening despite treatment
- Anticipation or experience of a significant interpersonal loss or psychosocial stressor (e.g., divorce, financial loss, legal problems, personal shame or humiliation)
- Onset of a physical illness (particularly if life threatening, disfiguring, or associated with severe pain or loss of executive functioning)

---

2. Specifically inquire about suicidal thoughts, plans, and behaviors.

Refer to Table 2, p. 187, for specific issues to address.

Elicit the presence or absence of suicidal ideation.
- Address the patient's feelings about living with questions such as "How does life seem to you at this point?" or "Have you ever felt that life was not worth living?" or "Did you ever wish you could go to sleep and just not wake up?"
- Focus on the nature, frequency, extent, and timing of suicidal thoughts, and consider their interpersonal, situational, and symptomatic context.
- Speak with family members or friends to determine whether they have observed behavior (e.g., recent purchase of a gun) or have been privy to thoughts that suggest suicidal ideation.
- If the patient is intoxicated with alcohol or other substances when initially interviewed, the patient's suicidality will need to be reassessed at a later time.

2. Specifically inquire about suicidal thoughts, plans, and behaviors (continued).

Elicit the presence or absence of a suicide plan.
- Probe for detailed information about specific plans for suicide and any steps that have been taken toward enacting those plans.
- Determine the patient's belief about the lethality of the method, which may be as important as the actual lethality of the method.
- Determine the conditions under which the patient would consider suicide (e.g., divorce, going to jail, housing loss) and estimate the likelihood that such a plan will be formed or acted on in the near future.
- Inquire about the presence of a firearm in the home or workplace. If a firearm is present, discuss with the patient or a significant other the importance of restricting access to, securing, or removing this and other weapons.

Assess the patient's degree of suicidality, including suicidal intent and lethality of plan.
Determine motivation for suicide, seriousness and extent of the patient's aim to die, associated behaviors or planning for suicide, and lethality of the method.

Recognize that suicide assessment scales have very low predictive values and do not provide reliable estimates of suicide risk.
Nonetheless, they may be useful in developing a thorough line of questioning about suicide or in opening communication with the patient.

TABLE 2. Questions That May Be Helpful in Inquiring About Specific Aspects of Suicidal Thoughts, Plans, and Behaviors

---

Begin with questions that address the patient's feelings about living:
- Have you ever felt that life was not worth living?
- Did you ever wish you could go to sleep and just not wake up?

Follow up with specific questions that ask about thoughts of death, self-harm, or suicide:
- Is death something you've thought about recently?
- Have things ever reached the point that you've thought of harming yourself?

For individuals who have thoughts of self-harm or suicide, ask:
- How often have those thoughts occurred (including frequency, obsessional quality, controllability)?
- How likely do you think it is that you will act on them in the future?
- What do you envision happening if you actually killed yourself (e.g., escape, reunion with significant other, rebirth, reactions of others)?
- Have you made a specific plan to harm or kill yourself? (If so, what does the plan include?)

For individuals who have attempted suicide or engaged in self-damaging action(s), parallel questions to those in the previous section can address the prior attempt(s). Additional questions can be asked in general terms or can refer to the specific method used and may include:
- Can you describe what happened (e.g., circumstances, precipitants, view of future, use of alcohol or other substances, method, intent, seriousness of injury)?
- What did you think would happen (e.g., going to sleep versus injury versus dying, getting a reaction out of a particular person)?
- Did you receive treatment afterward (e.g., medical versus psychiatric, emergency department versus inpatient versus outpatient)?

For individuals with repeated suicidal thoughts or attempts, ask:
- About how often have you tried to harm (or kill) yourself?
- When was the most recent time?
- Can you describe your thoughts at the time that you were thinking most seriously about suicide?

For individuals with psychosis, ask specifically about hallucinations and delusions:
- Have you ever done what the voices ask you to do? (What led you to obey the voices? If you tried to resist them, what made it difficult?)
- Have there been times when the voices told you to hurt or kill yourself? (How often? What happened?)
- Are there things that you've been feeling guilty about or blaming yourself for?

Consider assessing the patient's potential to harm others in addition to him- or herself:
- Are there others who you think may be responsible for what you're experiencing (e.g., persecutory ideas, passivity experiences)? Are you having any thoughts of harming them?
- Are there other people you would want to die with you?
- Are there others who you think would be unable to go on without you?

Questions are selected from Table 3 of APA's *Practice Guideline for the Assessment and Treatment of Patients With Suicidal Behaviors.* See that table for additional questions.

3. Establish a multiaxial diagnosis.

Note all current or past axis I or axis II diagnoses, including those that may currently be in remission.

Identify physical illnesses (axis III), since such diagnoses may also be associated with an increased risk of suicide.

Record psychosocial stressors (axis IV), which may be either acute or chronic. Consider the perceived importance of the life event for the individual patient.

Assess the patient's baseline and current levels of functioning (axis V).

4. Estimate suicide risk.

Identify factors that may increase or decrease the patient's level of risk.
- The presence of a psychiatric disorder is the most significant risk factor.
- Medical illness is also associated with increased likelihood of suicide. See Table 3, p. 189, for specific medical conditions that have been associated with increased risk.
- See Table 3 for additional factors that increase risk and Table 4 (p. 190) for protective effects.
- Almost all psychiatric disorders have been shown to increase suicide risk (Table 5, p. 190).

TABLE 3. Factors Associated With Increased Risk for Suicide

Suicidal thoughts/behaviors
- Suicidal ideas (current or previous)
- Suicidal plans (current or previous)
- Suicide attempts (including aborted or interrupted attempts)
- Lethality of suicidal plans or attempts
- Suicidal intent

Psychiatric diagnoses
- Major depressive disorder
- Bipolar disorder (primarily in depressive or mixed episodes)
- Schizophrenia
- Anorexia nervosa
- Alcohol use disorder
- Other substance use disorders
- Cluster B personality disorders (particularly borderline personality disorder)
- Comorbidity of axis I and/or axis II disorders

Physical illnesses
- Diseases of the nervous system
  Multiple sclerosis
  Huntington's disease
  Brain and spinal cord injury
  Seizure disorders
- Malignant neoplasms
- HIV/AIDS
- Peptic ulcer disease
- Chronic obstructive pulmonary disease, especially in men
- Chronic hemodialysis-treated renal failure
- Systemic lupus erythematosus
- Pain syndromes
- Functional impairment

Psychosocial features
- Recent lack of social support (including living alone)
- Unemployment
- Drop in socioeconomic status
- Poor relationship with family[a]
- Domestic partner violence[b]
- Recent stressful life event

Childhood traumas
- Sexual abuse
- Physical abuse

Genetic and familial effects
- Family history of suicide (particularly in first-degree relatives)
- Family history of mental illness, including substance use disorders

Psychological features
- Hopelessness
- Psychic pain[a]
- Severe or unremitting anxiety
- Panic attacks
- Shame or humiliation[a]
- Psychological turmoil[a]
- Decreased self-esteem[a]
- Extreme narcissistic vulnerability[a]
- Behavioral features
- Impulsiveness
- Aggression, including violence against others
- Agitation

Cognitive features
- Loss of executive function[b]
- Thought constriction (tunnel vision)
- Polarized thinking
- Closed-mindedness

Demographic features
- Male gender[c]
- Widowed, divorced, or single marital status, particularly for men
- Elderly age group (age group with greatest proportionate risk for suicide)
- Adolescent and young adult age groups (age groups with highest numbers of suicides)
- White race
- Gay, lesbian, or bisexual orientation[b]

Additional features
- Access to firearms
- Substance intoxication (in the absence of a formal substance use disorder diagnosis)
- Unstable or poor therapeutic relationship[a]

[a]Association with increased rate of suicide is based on clinical experience rather than formal research evidence.
[b]Associated with increased rate of suicide attempts, but no evidence is available on suicide rates per se.
[c]For suicide attempts, females have increased risk, compared with males.

TABLE 4. **Factors Associated With Protective Effects for Suicide**

- Children in the home[a]
- Sense of responsibility to family[b]
- Pregnancy
- Religiosity
- Life satisfaction
- Reality testing ability[b]
- Positive coping skills[b]
- Positive problem-solving skills[b]
- Positive social support
- Positive therapeutic relationship[b]

[a]Except among those with postpartum psychosis or mood disorder.
[b]Association with decreased rate of suicide is based on clinical experience rather than formal research evidence.

TABLE 5. **Risk of Suicide in Persons With Previous Suicide Attempts and Psychiatric Disorders[a]**

Condition	Number of Studies	Standardized Mortality Ratio (SMR)[b]	Annual Suicide Rate (%)	Estimated Lifetime Suicide Rate (%)
Previous suicide attempts	9	38.4	0.549	27.5
Psychiatric disorders				
Eating disorders	15	23.1		
Major depression	23	20.4	0.292	14.6
Sedative abuse	3	20.3		
Mixed drug abuse	4	19.2	0.275	14.7
Bipolar disorder	15	15.0	0.310	15.5
Opioid abuse	10	14.0		
Dysthymia	9	12.1	0.173	8.6
Obsessive-compulsive disorder	3	11.5	0.143	8.2
Panic disorder	9	10.0	0.160	7.2
Schizophrenia	38	8.45	0.121	6.0
Personality disorders	5	7.08	0.101	5.1
Alcohol abuse	35	5.86	0.084	4.2
Pediatric psychiatric disorders	11	4.73		
Cannabis abuse	1	3.85		
Neuroses	8	3.72		
Mental retardation	5	0.88		

[a]Based on a meta-analysis of 249 reports published between 1966 and 1993 (Harris EC, Barraclough B: "Suicide as an Outcome for Mental Disorders: A Meta-Analysis." *British Journal of Psychiatry* 170:205–228, 1997). Table adapted with permission.
[b]The SMR is the ratio of the observed mortality to the expected mortality and approximates the risk of mortality resulting from suicide in the presence of a particular condition. For the general population, the value of the SMR is 1.0, with an annual suicide rate of 0.014% per year and a lifetime rate of 0.72%.

B. Psychiatric Management

1. Establish and maintain a therapeutic alliance.

- Suicidal ideation and behaviors can be explored and addressed within the context of a cooperative doctor-patient relationship, with the ultimate goal of reducing suicide risk.
- Taking responsibility for a patient's care is not the same as taking responsibility for the patient's life.

2. Attend to the patient's safety.

For patients in emergency or inpatient settings, consider ordering observation on a one-to-one basis or by continuous closed-circuit television monitoring until an assessment of risk can be completed or if the patient is deemed to be at significant suicide risk.

Remove potentially hazardous items from the patient's room (if inpatient), and secure the patient's belongings.

Consider screening patients for potentially dangerous items by searching patients or scanning them with metal detectors.

3. Determine a treatment setting.

Treat in the setting that is least restrictive yet most likely to prove safe and effective (Table 6, p. 193).

Take into consideration the estimated suicide risk and the potential for dangerousness to others.

Reevaluate the optimal treatment setting and the patient's ability to benefit from a different level of care on an ongoing basis throughout the course of treatment.

4. Develop a plan of treatment.

Consider potential beneficial and adverse effects of each option along with information about the patient's preferences.

Address substance use disorders.

Provide more intense follow-up in the early stages of treatment to provide support and to rapidly institute treatment.

Review with outpatients guidelines for managing exacerbations of suicidal tendencies or other symptoms that may occur between scheduled sessions.

TABLE 6. Guidelines for Selecting a Treatment Setting for Patients at Risk for Suicide or Suicidal Behaviors

	Admission is generally indicated	Admission may be necessary	Release from emergency department with follow-up recommendations may be possible	Outpatient treatment may be more beneficial than hospitalization
After a suicide attempt or aborted suicide attempt . . .		Yes		
And patient is psychotic	Yes			
And attempt was violent, near-lethal, or premeditated	Yes			
And precautions were taken to avoid rescue or discovery	Yes			
And persistent plan and/or intent is present	Yes			
And distress is increased or patient regrets surviving	Yes			
And patient is male and older than age 45 years, especially with new onset of psychiatric illness or suicidal thinking	Yes			
And patient has limited family and/or social support, including lack of stable living situation	Yes			
And current impulsive behavior, severe agitation, poor judgment, or refusal of help is evident	Yes			
And patient has change in mental status with a metabolic, toxic, infectious, or other etiology requiring further workup in a structured setting	Yes			

TABLE 6. Guidelines for Selecting a Treatment Setting for Patients at Risk for Suicide or Suicidal Behaviors (continued)

	Admission is generally indicated	Admission may be necessary	Release from emergency department with follow-up recommendations may be possible	Outpatient treatment may be more beneficial than hospitalization
In the absence of a suicide attempt but in the presence of suicidal ideation . . .			Yes	
With specific plan with high lethality	Yes			
With high suicidal intent	Yes			
With psychosis		Yes		
With major psychiatric disorder		Yes		
With past attempts, particularly if medically serious		Yes		
With possibly contributing medical condition (e.g., acute neurological disorder, cancer, infection)		Yes		
With lack of response to or inability to cooperate with partial hospital or outpatient treatment		Yes		
With need for supervised setting for medication trial or ECT		Yes		
With need for skilled observation, clinical tests, or diagnostic assessments that require a structured setting		Yes		
With limited family and/or social support, including lack of stable living situation		Yes		
With lack of an ongoing clinician-patient relationship or lack of access to timely outpatient follow-up		Yes		

TABLE 6. Guidelines for Selecting a Treatment Setting for Patients at Risk for Suicide or Suicidal Behaviors (continued)

	Admission is generally indicated	Admission may be necessary	Release from emergency department with follow-up recommendations may be possible	Outpatient treatment may be more beneficial than hospitalization
In the absence of a suicide attempt but in the presence of suicidal ideation . . . (continued)				
But suicidality is a reaction to precipitating events (e.g., exam failure, relationship difficulties), particularly if the patient's view of situation has changed since coming to emergency department			Yes	
But plan/method and intent have low lethality			Yes	
But patient has stable and supportive living situation			Yes	
But patient is able to cooperate with recommendations for follow-up, with treater contacted, if possible, if patient is currently in treatment			Yes	
But without prior medically serious attempts, and if a safe and supportive living situation is available and outpatient psychiatric care is ongoing				Yes
In the absence of suicide attempts or reported suicidal ideation/plan/intent . . .				
But evidence from the psychiatric evaluation and/or history from others suggests a high level of suicide risk and a recent acute increase in risk		Yes		Yes

5. Coordinate care and collaborate with other clinicians.

Establish clear role definitions, regular communication among team members, and advance planning for management of crises.

Communicate with other caregivers, including other physicians providing treatment for significant general medical conditions or other mental health professionals who may be providing therapy. Establish guidelines for contact in the event of a significant clinical change.

6. Promote adherence to the treatment plan.

Establish a positive physician-patient relationship.

Create an atmosphere in which the patient feels free to discuss positive or negative aspects of the treatment process.

7. Provide education to the patient and family.

8. Reassess safety and suicide risk.

► Repeat suicide assessments over time, because of the waxing and waning nature of suicidality (see Table 1, p. 185, for settings and circumstances).

► Repeat suicide assessments in inpatient settings at critical stages of treatment (e.g., with a change in level of privilege, abrupt change in mental state, and before discharge).

► Reassess suicidality if the patient was intoxicated with alcohol or other substances when initially interviewed.

9. Monitor psychiatric status and response to treatment.

• Monitoring is especially important during the early phases of treatment, since some medications may take several weeks to provide therapeutic benefit.
• An early increase in suicide risk may occur as depressive symptoms begin to lift but before they are fully resolved.

10. Obtain consultation, if indicated.

• Consultation may be of help in monitoring and addressing countertransference issues.
• Consultation may be important in affirming the appropriateness of the treatment plan or suggesting other possible therapeutic approaches.

C. Specific Treatment Modalities

1. Somatic Therapies

The strong association between depressive disorders and suicide supports the use of **antidepressants.**

Long-term maintenance treatment with **lithium salts** in patients with recurring bipolar disorder and major depressive disorder is associated with substantial reductions in risk of both suicide and suicide attempts.

There is no established evidence of a reduced risk of suicidal behavior with any other **"mood-stabilizing" anticonvulsant agents.**

Reductions in the rates of suicide attempts and suicide have been reported in specific studies of patients with schizophrenia treated with **clozapine.** Other first- and second-generation **antipsychotics** may also reduce suicide risk, particularly in highly agitated patients.

Because anxiety is a significant and modifiable risk factor for suicide, use of **antianxiety agents** may have the potential to decrease this risk. However, **benzodiazepines** occasionally disinhibit aggressive and dangerous behaviors and enhance impulsivity, particularly in patients with borderline personality disorder.

ECT may reduce suicidal ideation, at least in the short term.

2. Psychotherapies

Clinical consensus suggests that **psychosocial interventions** and **specific psychotherapeutic approaches** are of benefit.

D. Documentation and Risk Management

1. General Issues Specific to Suicide

- It is crucial for the suicide risk assessment to be documented in the medical record.
- See Table 7, p. 200, for general risk management considerations.

2. Suicide Prevention Contracts

- Reliance on a suicide prevention contract may falsely lower clinical vigilance without altering the patient's suicidal state.
- If a suicide prevention contract is used, a patient's unwillingness to commit to the contract mandates reassessment of the therapeutic alliance and the patient's level of suicide risk.
- Suicide prevention contracts are not recommended in emergency settings; with newly admitted and unknown inpatients; with agitated, psychotic, or impulsive patients; or when the patient is under the influence of an intoxicating substance.

TABLE 7. General Risk Management and Documentation Considerations in the Assessment and Management of Patients at Risk for Suicide

Good collaboration, communication, and alliance between clinician and patient

Careful and attentive documentation, including:
- Risk assessments
- Record of decision-making processes
- Descriptions of changes in treatment
- Record of communications with other clinicians
- Record of telephone calls from patients or family members
- Prescription log or copies of actual prescriptions
- Medical records of previous treatment, if available, particularly treatment related to past suicide attempts

Critical junctures for documentation:
- At first psychiatric assessment or admission
- With occurrence of any suicidal behavior or ideation
- Whenever there is any noteworthy clinical change
- For inpatients, before increasing privileges or giving passes and before discharge

Monitoring issues of transference and countertransference in order to optimize clinical judgment

Consultation, a second opinion, or both should be considered when necessary

Careful termination (with appropriate documentation)

Firearms:
- If present, document instructions given to the patient and significant others
- If absent, document as a pertinent negative

Planning for coverage

3. Communication With Significant Others

If a patient is (or is likely to become) dangerous to him- or herself or to others and will not consent to interventions intended to reduce those risks, the psychiatrist is justified in attenuating confidentiality to the extent needed to address the safety of the patient and others.

4. Management of Suicide in One's Practice

- If a patient dies by suicide, ensure that his or her records are complete.
- Conversations with family members can be appropriate and can allay grief and assist devastated family members in obtaining help.
- In speaking with survivors, care must be exercised not to reveal confidential information about the patient and not to make self-incriminating or self-exonerating statements.

5. Mental Health Interventions for Surviving Family and Friends After a Suicide

Suggest psychiatric intervention to family members and friends shortly after the death to reduce their risk for psychiatric impairment.

Consider referring surviving family members and friends to a survivor support group.